PAIN MANAGEMENT

Edited by **Milica Prostran**

Pain Management
http://dx.doi.org/10.5772/61605
Edited by Milica Prostran

Contributors

Serbulent Gokhan Beyaz, Havva Sayhan, Wen-Long Hu, Hyun Jeong Park, Hwa Young Jung, Suleyman Deniz, Omer Bakal, Gokhan Inangil, Anna Rutkowska, Grażyna Skotnicka-Klonowicz, Linda Papa, Ivan Samcam, Shahnawaz Anwer, Ahmad Alghadir

Published by InTech

Janeza Trdine 9, 51000 Rijeka, Croatia

Publishing Process Manager Ana Simcic
Technical Editor InTech DTP team
Cover InTech Design team

First published May, 2016
Printed in Croatia

Additional hard copies can be obtained from orders@intechopen.com

Pain Management , Edited by Milica Prostran
p. cm.
Print ISBN 978-953-51-2413-9
Online ISBN 978-953-51-2414-6

For EU product safety concerns:
IN TECH d.o.o., Prolaz Marije Krucifikse Kozulić 3, 51000 Rijeka, Croatia,
info@intechopen.com or visit our website at intechopen.com.

Meet the editor

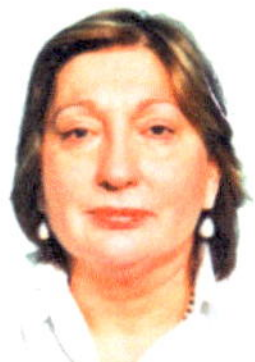

Professor Milica Prostran, MD, PhD, graduated from the School of Medicine, University of Belgrade, Serbia. She obtained a Master of Science degree in cardiology and a PhD in Pharmacology. Professor Prostran, the president of the Pharmaceutical Medicine Section of the Serbian Medical Association, is the Head of Master course in Pharmaceutical Medicine. She is a member of several important governmental bodies. She published over 180 in extenso papers in peer-reviewed journals indexed in CC/SCI, as well as over 50 chapters in books. Professor Prostran serves as a member (and referee) of the Editorial Board of several highly respected international journals as well as several national scientific and professional journals.

Contents

Preface IX

Chapter 1 **Acute Pain Management in the Emergency Department 1**
Ivan Samcam MD and Linda Papa MD, MSc

Chapter 2 **The Quality of Prehospital Medical Care Provided to Children with Traumatic Injuries 27**
Anna Rutkowska and Grażyna Skotnicka-Klonowicz

Chapter 3 **Managing Pain with Laser Acupuncture 49**
Szu-Ying Wu, Chun-En Kuo, Yu-Chiang Hung and Wen-Long Hu

Chapter 4 **Pain Management of Herpes Zoster 61**
Hwa Young Jung and Hyun Jeong Park

Chapter 5 **Pain Management in Knee Osteoarthritis 81**
Shahnawaz Anwer and Ahmad Alghadir

Chapter 6 **Application of Radiofrequency in Pain Management 95**
Suleyman Deniz, Omer Bakal and Gokhan Inangil

Chapter 7 **Epiduroscopy (Epidural Endoscopy) 115**
Havva Sayhan and Serbulent Gokhan Beyaz

Preface

This book *Pain Management* has 7 chapters, from more than 15 authors from different countris (Korea, Poland, Saudi Arabia, Taiwan, Turkey and USA) of the world and one editor, Professor Milica Prostran. Professor Prostran, MD, PhD is a pharmacologist as well as a clinical pharmacologist with subspeciality in clinical pharmacology - pharmacotherapy. This was due to her experience with publishing in respected international journals: she published over 180 in *extenso* papers in peer review international journals indexed in *CC/SCI,* and over 50 chapters in various books, Professor Prostran has compiled a collection of manuscripts (see List of her selected references at the end of this text).

Topics covered in *Pain Management* vary among *Acute pain management in the emergency department, The quality of prehospital care give to children with traumatic injuries, Managing pain with laser acupuncture, Pain management of Herpes Zoster, Pain management in knee osteoarthritis, Application of radiofrequency in pain management to Epiduroscopy (Epidural endoscopy).*

The most common complaint in the Emergency Department is pain. According to authors of this chapter (Samcam and Papa), "objectively assessing and documenting a patient's pain is the key to determining treatment. The approach to a patient with acute pain requires an experienced clinician who is awere of the pharmacology of analgesics and anesthetics, contraindications, precautions, side effects, administration methods and monitoring requirements."

Rutkowska et al. concluded among other things that "The management of the child with an injury in the Lodzkie region (in Poland) is unsatisfactory. Despite the training of physicians, nureses and paramedics in the management of paediatric injuries, the lack of analgesic provision is still encountered in almost half of patients, irregularities in transport immobilisation - in about 10% of the patients and irregularities in wound management and IV access provision - in isolated cases. In 1/4 of the cases, gaps in medical records were also noted."

Wu et al. presented a paper dealing with laser acupuncture, introduced clinically for the first time in the 1970s. They stated that "Laser acupuncture relieves pain through both anti-inflammatory and analgesic effects. No adverse effects or complications resulting from laser acupuncture were reported in the litarature. In the hands of an experienced physician, laser acupuncture can be a useful and safe method for pain management."

Jung and Park in their review focused on the treatment options available for management of patients with acute HZ *(Herpes Zoster)* and PHN (Post-Herpetic Neuralgia), while Anwer and Alghadir, stated that "Management of knee OA ofter requires a combination of pharmacologic and nonpharmacologic treatment approaches."

Deniz et al. stated "...the use of continuous and pulsed radiofrequency with a minimal invasive procedure for patients with chronic pain as an alternative to surgical treatment and it might be an additional option among nonsurgical treatment methods."

And, the last chapter deals with epidural endoscopy in detail. Sayhan and Beyaz concluded that "Incidence of complications is inversely proportional to professional skills of practitioner and the number of years of experience. It should be borne in mind, there are risk associated with medical procedures in the spinal region, even when it is performed properly and conscientiously."

The potential reader is shown the modern approach to pain management because the chapters deal at length and clearly with the topics.

I believe that this book *Pain Management* I edited with great pleasure and dedication will capture the attention of many readers, from medical students, practicing medical doctors as well as biomedical researchers. All of them need to deal with this extremely important field of treating pain. Additionally, I do believe that the answers they may find in *Pain Management* will make their practice easier. Also, the life of their patients will be considerably more pleasant, or at least more bearable.

Last but not least, I want to express my gratitude to Ms. Ana Simčić, publishing process manager from InTech for her constant help in editing this book.

List of Professor Milica Prostran selected references:

Vučković S, Prostran M, Ivanović M, Ristović Z, Stojanović R. Antinociceptive activity of the novel fentanyl analogue iso-carfentanyl in rats. Jpn J Pharmacol. 2000; 84: 188-95.

Mićović IV, Ivanović MD, Vučković SM, Prostran MŠ, Došen-Mićović Lj, Kiricojević VD. The synthesis and preliminary pharmacological evaluation of 4-methyl fentanyl. Boorg Med Chem Lett. 2000; 10:2011-4.

Vučković SM, Tomić MA, Stepanović-Petrović RM, Ugrešić N, Prostran MŠ, Bošković B. The effects of alpha2-adrenoceptor agents on anti-hyperalgesic effects of carbamazepine and oxcarbazepine in rat model of inflammatory pain. Pain. 2006; 25:10-9.

Tomić MA, Vučković SM, Stepanović-Petrović RM, Ugrešić ND, Prostran MŠ, Bošković B. Synergistic interactios between paracetamol and oxcarbazepine in somatic and visceral pain in rodents. Anesth Analg. 2010; 110: 1198-205.

Srebro DP, Vučković SM, Savić Vujović KR, Prostran MS. TRPA1, NMDA receptors and nitric oxide mediate mechanical hyperalgesia induced by local injection of magnesium sulfate into the rat hind paw. Physiol Behav. 2015; 139: 267-73.

Professor Milica Prostran MD PhD
Department of Pharmacology, Clinical Pharmacology And Toxicology
Faculty of Medicine, University of Belgrade
Belgrade
Serbia

Chapter 1

Acute Pain Management in the Emergency Department

Ivan Samcam MD and Linda Papa MD, MSc

Additional information is available at the end of the chapter

http://dx.doi.org/10.5772/62861

Abstract

The most common presenting complaint to the emergency department (emergency room) is pain. Unfortunately, pain is still undertreated in this setting. Literature has shown that treatment of pain not only improves patient satisfaction but also improves mood, decreases length of hospital stay, and decreases mortality. Various pharmacological options are available for treating acute pain, ranging from oral, intravenous, and intramuscular medications; topical agents; and peripheral nerve blocks. Objectively assessing and documenting a patient's pain is the key to determining treatment. The approach to a patient with acute pain requires an experienced clinician who is aware of the pharmacology of analgesics and anesthetics, contraindications, precautions, side effects, administration methods, and monitoring requirements.

This chapter briefly covers the pathophysiology of acute pain and the different treatment modalities available to the emergency physician.

Keywords: pain, acute, emergency, treatment, management

1. Introduction

1.1. Epidemiology

The most common presenting complaint to the emergency department (ED) room is pain. From 1996 to 2015, ED visits have risen over 46%, from 90.3 million to [1] 136 million [1, 2]. As emergency room visits continue to grow every year, so does the need to treat patients in pain. Roughly, 45% of ED visits involves either moderate or severe pain [3]. The most common pain-related chief complaints in descending order are chest pain, back pain, and headache. Furthermore, the most frequently ordered analgesics, both in the ED and at discharge, are acetaminophen (alone or in combination with hydrocodone), ketorolac, and ibuprofen [3].

1.2. Oligoanalgesia

Despite the trend in increasing ED visits of which the majority involves pain, pain is still undertreated in the ED. Oligoanalgesia is a term used to describe the inadequate treatment of pain and was first studied in a retrospective chart analysis in 1989 by Wilson and Pendleton [4]. In this study, a total of 198 patients were evaluated, and of those who received analgesics, 32% received less than optimal doses [5]. An additional retrospective study, done a few years later, revealed that only 30% of 401 patients treated for bone fractures received analgesics [6]. In a separate study, patients were surveyed after treatment in a fast-track area of the emergency room, and 60% of patients went home with more pain than they were willing to accept [7]. More recently, a prospective, multicenter study enrolled 842 patients (aged 8 years and older) across 20 US and Canadian EDs with presenting pain intensity scores of 4 or greater on an 11-point numerical rating scale and found that only 60% of patients received analgesics, and 74% of patients were discharged in moderate to severe pain. Furthermore, reassessments were uncommon, and analgesics were administered after lengthy delays (median, 90 minutes; range, 0–962 minutes) [8].

1.3. Why is treating pain important?

The Joint Commission on Accreditation of Hospitals Organization (JCAHO) has recommended that assessment and treatment of pain be improved. Moreover, patients expect to have their pain treated fairly quickly and to have it significantly reduced. Studies have shown that patients want their pain treated in less than half an hour, yet the mean time of treatment is at least 78 minutes [9]. Acknowledging and treating pain in the ED improves the rapport between physician and patient. Patients are more likely to characterize physicians who treat their pain as warm and friendly and inspire more confidence to discuss their private health concerns [10]. Inadequately treating pain can contribute to the development of comorbidities such as depression, hypertension, and immune system dysfunction [10].

There are numerous potential reasons for which pain is inadequately treated in the ED, such as concern of masking symptoms, poor communication between clinician and patient (language, cultural), lack of documentation and reassessment of pain, and fear of contributing to and causing addiction. One of the most cited reasons is the concern that analgesics, particularly opioids, may mask symptoms of a surgical abdomen. This concern has been refuted by a number of studies. A randomized double-controlled trial conducted in 2002 evaluated pain control in the diagnosis of appendicitis. Pain was adequately treated, and patients continued to have pain upon palpation on physical examination [11]. An additional study studied the surgeon's confidence in physical signs after administration of morphine to patients with appendicitis. Despite the morphine, these surgeons continued to illicit examination signs such as the obturator sign, Rovsing, and pain upon jumping [12]. Other physicians may argue that opioids may mask the intensity of pain allowing for the progression of the illness to complications such as perforation and formation of an intra-abdominal abscess. A systematic review of six randomized controlled trials evaluating the safety of opioid administration to children with acute abdominal pain showed no significant difference in the rate of perforation or abscess formation [13]

The concern over causing addiction plays an important role in oligoanalgesia in the ED. In 2012, health care providers wrote 259 million prescriptions for painkillers. This is equivalent to every American adult having a bottle of pills. Furthermore, each day, 46 people die from an overdose of prescription painkillers in the United States [14].

In 2007 the cost of prescription opioid abuse was estimate to be $56 billion dollars [15]. Those with a prior history of depression, anxiety, and substance use were most likely to have a propensity for prescription opioid abuse [16]. An additional study confirmed mental disease as risk factor for opioid abuse, as well as males, younger adults, and individuals with greater days of supply of prescription opioid abuse. Thus, the emergency physician must do a full history, including a psychiatric history, prior to considering opioids.

Screening programs not only elucidate a patient's past-filled prescriptions but can also give the physician an idea of the different pharmacies and health clinics the patient has gone to. This information gives the prescriber insight into any drug-seeking behavior and may change their propensity into prescribing a certain analgesic [17].

1.4. Documentation of pain

The effective management of acute pain in the ED requires appropriate assessment of the pain based on the patient's perception of pain using a validated pain scale. Additionally, reassessment of pain is essential to determine the effect of treatment. Pain has been described as a vital sign, and as such it should be documented in the initial assessment of a patient. Verbal pain scores (VPSs) may reveal those who are truly in pain but who may not voice their discomfort, as well as influence the physician to inquire about the patient's pain. One study revealed, that in patients who did not receive analgesics, 42% desired them, but only 31% voiced their concern [8]. A prospective study introducing VPSs in an ED revealed that of those trauma patients who had VPS scores documented, 60% received analgesics versus 33% in those who did not have a VPS score documented. Furthermore, those with higher VPS scores were more likely to receive analgesics [18]. ED crowding has been shown to increase time to analgesic administration and mortality [19]. The use of VPS in this setting may identify those individuals in need of quicker treatment.

2. Pathophysiology

Pain can be divided into acute and chronic, with acute pain being incited by a traumatic injury or pathologic condition. As the causative issue is addressed, acute pain is usually resolved. Acute pain is mediated through nociceptors, of which there are various types ranging from mechanical to thermoreceptors. These receptors are stimulated by chemical, thermal, or mechanical stimuli [20]. As these receptors are stimulated, sensory neurons transmit the stimulus through neuronal pathways made up of various peripheral nerve fibers. "First Pain," which is well localized and sharp, is modulated by Aδ-fibers. The second component of pain, or the slow phase, is conducted by C fibers and is characterized by dull and poorly localized pain [21].

All pain starts as acute pain; however, not all pain progresses to chronic pain. Acute pain becomes chronic when pain persists despite the resolution of the inciting event. There may be many causative factors that account for prolonged pain. Apart from the psychosocial influences on chronic pain development, physiologic factors that contribute to chronic pain include alterations in the spinal cord that occur when acute pain is inadequately treated. These changes lead to increased excitability, decreased inhibition, and reorganization of certain spinal tracts [22]. The time frame for defining chronic pain varies from 3 to 6 months of ongoing pain. However, some would argue that chronic pain is any pain that persists longer than the reasonably expected healing time for the involved tissues. It is also important to understand that an individual's perception of pain may be influenced by culture, previous painful experiences, beliefs, mood, and ability to cope.

2.1. Somatic and visceral pain

Somatic pain is made up of mostly A-fibers and is located in cutaneous tissues as well as deep tissues such as fascia, tendons, or bone. This pain is described as initially sharp and then as burning or throbbing. On the contrary, visceral pain is primarily composed of C f-fibers, and its primary afferent neuron endings are usually found in internal organs such as intestines, gonads, or heart [21]. For example, at presentation, pain from appendicitis may initially be poorly localized around the periumbilical site and characterized as dull, indicating primarily a visceral pain. However, as inflammation continues, the above fascia tissues become inflamed. At this point, pain is now located at the right lower quadrant and may be sharp. This later presentation of appendicitis is now primarily involving the somatic cutaneous nerves in the corresponding dermatome. Asking the patient to initially describe the pain may hint toward the initial causative pathologic condition. For instance, in a patient with sharp and clearly localized back pain, the causative agent may be musculoskeletal in nature. However, those with dull, achy, and poorly localized pain, back pain radiating to the groin may be due to an internal cause such as pyelonephritis or nephrolithiasis.

2.2. Neuronal pathway

The initiating stimulus of pain is conducted through these peripheral nerve fibers. There are a number of neuronal pathways through neuronal pathways, but the spinothalamic tract is the main pathway. These pathways converge into primary afferent neurons found in the dorsal root ganglion. Afferent neurons have two endings: one signaling the peripheral system and the second signaling second-order neurons in the dorsal horn. The second-order neurons' axons cross the midline of the spinal cord into the contralateral spinothalamic tract, where they ascend into the thalamus. Third-order neurons in the thalamus synapse with the second-order neurons and send signals to the post-central gyrus of the cerebral cortex [21]. As the nerve fibers ascend in the spinal cord, they organize into dorsolateral columns and anteromedial segments [20].

The dorsal columns and anterior medial segment are divided into different segments called laminae. This is done to organize the type of sensory information sent into each section [23]. Laminae 1 through 6 are located in the dorsal horn, 7 through 10 in the intermediate zone, and 8 though 9 in the anterior/ventral horn. The gray matter surrounding the central cord composes lamina 10. All afferent nerve activity is received in the dorsal horn. Specifically, lamina 1 receives mostly noxious stimuli from cutaneous tissues and deep somatic tissues. Visceral afferent fibers are transmitted to laminas 5 and 1. However, lamina 5 also receives somatic afferent fibers, and it is this convergence that leads to referred pain [21]. Lamina 2, or the substantia gelatinosa of Rolando, mediates the activity of pain and temperature afferent fibers. Next, lamina 3 and 4, known as the nucleus proprius, receive input from lamina 2 and also help regulate pain, temperature, as well as crude touch. Lamina 7 receives afferent input from muscle fibers and joints [24].

Furthermore, the spinothalamic tract is subdivided into a lateral and a medial tract. The lateral tract projects to the ventral posterolateral nucleus of the thalamus and carries fibers sensory input that transmits location, intensity, and duration of pain. The medial tract projects to the medial nucleus of the thalamus and mediates the emotional and autonomic aspects of pain. Collateral fibers from the spinothalamic tract are also projected to the RAS, or reticular activating system, as well as the hypothalamus [21]. These collateral fibers may be responsible for the arousal aspect of pain.

2.3. Modulation of pain

Descending tracts originating from the midbrain and medulla feed into the spinal cord through the dorsolateral funiculus, modulating pain [20]. For example, stimulation of the periaqueductal gray, through projections from the spinothalamic tract, provides widespread analgesia in humans [25, 26]. One investigator noted that stimulation of the periaqueductal gray leads to analgesia with such significance that one could perform an exploratory laparotomy without any chemical anesthesia [26, 27]. Furthermore, these tracts involve transmitters such as norepinephrine, serotonin, and opiates [20]. TCAs and SSRIs through these neurotransmitters have been shown in various studies to significantly reduce chronic pain, regardless of the patient's psychosocial status. A meta-analysis found there is no difference in pain relief from the use of these medications in the absence or presence of depression, and the size of analgesia is not significantly different in the presence or absence of anti-depressant effect [28].

Additional modulation of pain can be seen through the endorphin system. This system consists of neurons that secrete three types of opioids beta-endorphin, net- and leu-enkaphalins, and dynorphins. These chemicals act on the mu, delta, and kappa receptors modulating pain relief [20].

3. Common analgesic agents used in the emergency department

3.1. Opioids

Opioid prescriptions for the management of non-cancer pain have increased over the last 10–20 years. Concerns of opioid dependence and toxicity, such as respiratory depression, have led to the under-dosing of these agents in the ED and the use of other less effective analgesic agents.

3.1.1. Mechanism

The term opioid refers to natural and synthetic substances that act at one of the three main opioid receptor systems (mu, kappa, delta). They can have analgesic and central nervous system (CNS) depressant effects as well as the potential to cause euphoria. The majority of opioids used clinically target μ-opioid (mu) receptors. These receptors mediate analgesia as well as common side effects such as euphoria, constipation, and respiratory depression [29]. One exception is the combination of agonist–antagonist agents such as buprenorphine. Another less commonly targeted receptor is the **κ**-opioid (kappa) receptor, which is important in regulating GI motility and dysphoria. The other endorphin receptors may regulate neuropathic pain, as we all as spinal anesthesia.

3.1.2. Morphine

One of the most commonly used opioids in the ED is morphine. It is considered safe and effective in the monitored setting in the ED [29].

Side effects can range from hypotension, pruritus, nausea, vomiting, and respiratory depression. It is believed that some of these side effects may be due to the destabilization of mast cells that lead to the release of histamine. Respiratory depression is caused by desensitization of the medulla to carbon dioxide, through opioids binding to the mu receptor. The cardiovascular effects of opioids are mediated centrally at the central vagal nucleus and, in the case of morphine, directly into the sinoatrial node. Within the gastrointestinal system, opioids delay gastric emptying and cause constipation [29]. There appears to be no significant differences in side effects between dosages of 0.1 mg/kg and 0.15 mg/kg.

Weight-based dosing for morphine is not necessary in obese patients. A prospective observational study in the ED revealed that patient's weight was not predictive of pain reduction [30]. Thus one should start with the recommended dose of 0.1 mg/kg if side effects are of concern; however, one should be ready to rebolus in 5–15 minutes as studies have revealed this initial dosing is inadequate. A prospective cohort study of 119 patients revealed that 67% of patients who received 0.1 mg/kg of morphine stated less than 50% reduction of pain 30 minutes later [31]. A later study evaluating trauma patients revealed that a dose of 0.15 mg/kg when compared to 0.1 mg/kg significantly reduces pain without any significant difference in adverse events [32].

In the setting of trauma, hypotension may reduce tissue perfusion in patients with significant blood loss. However, in a randomized controlled study in acute trauma patients, hypotension only occurred in 10% of patients who received morphine [32]. A study investigating the use of morphine in the pre-hospital setting in ST segment elevation myocardial infarction patients found no worsening of in-hospital complications or 1-year mortality [33]. The cancer literature has also shown the value and safety of morphine infusions for pain control [34].

3.1.3. Hydromorphone

Hydromorphone is a semisynthetic derivative of morphine that is seven times more potent than morphine. Despite the increased potency, studies have shown that nurses who are concerned about side effects may give a lower dose of morphine versus hydromorphone since the "total milligrams" given in hydromorphone is less when compared to an equal analgesic dose of morphine [35]. Despite the dosing difference, hydromorphone appears to offer better pain control. In a retrospective study involving the use of patient-controlled analgesia (PCA) with either morphine or hydromorphone, more patients receiving morphine required rescue analgesia due to initial inadequate pain control [36].

Pruritus occurs less frequently with hydromorphone. Hydromorphone is conjugated by the liver to hydromorphone-3-glucoronide, an inactive metabolite. However, morphine's metabolite is active, and as a result, hydromorphone is better tolerated [20]. With regard to adverse effects, hydromorphone has not been shown to have an increased risk, and its use does not necessitate increased naloxone administration [37].

3.1.4. Fentanyl

When pain relief is needed quickly for acute severe pain, such as in trauma, fentanyl may be of use. Its time of onset is 1–2 minutes and lasts typically about 30 minutes [20]. The initial IV dose is 1.5 μg/kg, and it has the advantage of a short half-life. This is particularly useful if serial examinations are needed. Fentanyl causes minimal histamine release, making it ideal in patients in whom blood pressure must be maintained. For example, in severe traumatic brain injury patients, in whom MAP must be kept above 80 to maintain cerebral perfusion pressure, and must be examined serially, fentanyl may be a useful analgesic. The safety profile is favorable, particularly in the pre-hospital setting. A retrospective chart review of 2,129 patients transported by Emergency Medical Services revealed that fentanyl affected vital signs in less than 1% of patients [38]. Despite its favorable hemodynamic profile, fentanyl may cause chest wall rigidity when given in doses above 15 μg/ kg leading to inadequate ventilation. This is a rare complication and can be remedied through neuromuscular blockade or naloxone [39, 40].

3.2. Non-opioid medications

Non-opioid analgesics include acetaminophen, non-selective nonsteroidal anti-inflammatory drugs (NSAIDs), and cyclooxygenase 2 (COX-2) inhibitors. NSAIDs and COX 2 inhibitors have anti-inflammatory properties.

3.2.1. *Acetaminophen*

A common over-the-counter analgesic for mild to moderate pain is acetaminophen (para-acetylaminophenol) or paracetamol (in Europe). Its mechanism of action is through the inhibition of prostaglandin endoperoxide H_2 synthase and cyclooxygenase activity [20, 41]. Its central anti-pyretic effect is of great use when fever needs to be reduced. It has been shown to have good analgesic effects; however, acetaminophen is not anti-inflammatory. Systematic reviews have shown that acetaminophen can significantly reduce pain; however, it may be less effective than NSAIDs in conditions such as back pain and osteoarthritis [42–44]. Acetaminophen can also be combined with opioid medications to reduce the amount of opioid needed. However, concerns about unintentional acetaminophen overdose have led to combination drug products with more than 325 mg acetaminophen per tablet to be withdrawn from the market. Acetaminophen overdose can lead to severe hepatotoxicity and should be used cautiously in patients with chronic alcohol use or liver disease.

Intravenous acetaminophen is being studied for acute pain such as in acute traumatic limb injuries [45] or rib fractures [46] or in postoperative patients [47, 48]. It has also been shown to reduce the need for rescue pain medications such as opioids [49, 50].

3.2.2. *Nonsteroidal anti-inflammatory drugs*

NSAIDs provide analgesia for mild to moderate pain and also work synergistically when paired with opioids. They work through the inhibition of cyclooxygenase by decreasing the production of prostaglandins and prostacyclins, primarily cyclooxygenase 1 (COX-1) and COX-2. COX-1 mediates platelet aggregation and maintenance of gastrointestinal mucosal integrity. By contrast, COX-2 generates prostaglandins that mediate pain and inflammation [29]. The different NSAIDs can be either selective COX-2 inhibitors or non-selective, thus differing in their side-effect profile. There are many NSAIDs to choose from, but there is little literature showing improved efficacy of one NSAID over another.

Main adverse side effects of NSAIDs include gastrointestinal insult, renal insult, inhibition of platelets, cardiovascular effects, and anaphylaxis. Renal failure is caused by the decreased production of prostaglandins, which aid in afferent glomerular arteriole vasodilation. NSAIDs contribute to arteriolar vasoconstriction, leading to decreased renal perfusion pressure and decreased glomerular filtration rates [51]. This is worsened by dehydration. As selectivity of COX inhibition increases, the renal effects decrease. NSAIDs such as ketorolac and diclofenac have fewer effects on the kidney than naproxen or ibuprofen [51, 52].

The most common side effect of NSAIDs is gastrointestinal injury, such as bleeding or dyspepsia and gastric ulceration. Patients who are at high risk for peptic ulcer disease or its complications, such as the elderly, those with bleeding diathesis, or patients on glucocorticoids, have a relative contraindication to the use of an NSAID. Each NSAID has variability in the risk of gastrointestinal injury it poses. This is due to the selectivity of COX-1 inhibition, so that the relative risk of for ibuprofen is 2.6, while the relative risk for ketorolac is 14.5 [51, 53].

Various studies have shown that COX-2 inhibition is related to increased cardiovascular risk. This is believed to be the result of decreased prostacyclin (prostaglandin I_2) and increased thromboxane A_2. The effects lead to hypertension, accelerated atherogenesis, and increased thrombotic response to plaque rupture [54]. Myocardial infarction was found to be increased in this class of NSAIDs, resulting in the discontinuation of rofecoxib [55, 56]. Furthermore, it has been shown that specific COX-2 inhibitors may also further inhibit renal perfusion and lead to decreased sodium excretion, which may further worsen congestive heart failure and renal function [57, 58]. Due to COX-2 specific inhibitor side-effect profile and no proven increased efficacy over non-selective NSAIDs, there is minimal to no advantage in using this class in the ED.

There has been no proven efficacy over one type of NSAID, including the route of administration such as intra-muscular versus oral [29, 59, 60]. One should select a particular NSAID based on its side-effect profile and the route of administration that is the most feasible for the patient. Furthermore, prior to using NSAIDs, one must also take into consideration that this class of pharmaceuticals is most useful when used in pain mediated by prostaglandins or inflammation, not in other situations such as neuropathic pain. For instance, NSAID, particularly ketorolac, has been shown to significantly reduce pain in renal colic, and has similar efficacy in pain reduction as morphine [61]. When used in combination, opiates and NSAIDs may reduce the need of additional doses of analgesic rescue therapy in renal colic and have greater pain efficacy than either drug used alone [62]. In acute lower back pain, NSAIDs have been shown to significantly reduce pain and improve daily function [63]. The addition of opioids in this setting of pain was not proven to be more effective than NSAIDs alone [64].

3.2.3. Antispasmotics (muscle relaxants)

Muscle relaxants have been used by the physicians with the intention of alleviating musculoskeletal pain. However, data on this class of medications have produced mixed results since their action may be more the result of sedation rather than muscle relaxation. A systematic review, evaluating the effectiveness of cyclobenzaprine in lower back pain, revealed short-term improvement of pain at 7 days. However, there was no improvement of pain at 14 days, and there was no statistical difference when compared to diazepam [65]. Furthermore, in a second review evaluating the effectiveness of muscle relaxants in neck pain, there was no difference when compared to placebo at 2 weeks [66].

When compared to NSAIDs, muscle relaxants have been shown to have no significant difference in pain relief or improvement in daily function. Moreover, there is little to no added benefit when using muscle relaxants together with NSAIDs [64, 67]. Given the limited data on muscle relaxants, one should consider the side effects. Major side effects range from drowsiness, dizziness, dry mouth as well as other anticholinergic effects. These medications should only be prescribed for short-term use, given the limited data regarding efficacy past 1 week. In addition, one should refrain from prescribing these medications in the elderly, as they are at higher risk of falls and delirium.

3.2.4. Topical analgesics

There are various topical agents ranging from patches, gel, sprays to creams, which may aid in relieving pain. They appear to have several potential advantages over systemic drugs such as delivery at the site of injury, lower levels of systemic absorption, and fewer systemic effects. Although systemic side effects are not as frequent as oral formulations, significant systemic concentration can be achieved by topical application.

Often, these agents have similar efficacy to their oral preparations. For example, a randomized controlled trial comparing a gel preparation of ibuprofen versus oral tablets revealed comparable improvement in patient's pain and functional status at 2 weeks [68]. Topical agents often have fewer side effects than their oral counterparts, and most adverse events are primarily cutaneous in nature such as rashes or pruritus. Decreased adverse events may be due to lower bioavailability in the plasma [69, 70]. Many factors may influence the penetration of the topical agent into the local site. Variability in an individual's skin properties such as the thickness of stratum corneum may be a limiting factor. Furthermore, the agent must be lipophilic and water-soluble [71]. Local site pH, such as acidity in a local cellulitis, may also limit penetration of the agent.

Topical NSAIDs have been shown to have rare incidences of gastrointestinal adverse events such as ulcer formation, as opposed to oral formulations [69]. Topical diclofenac and ibuprofen have been shown to be effective in acute soft tissue injuries, such as ankle sprains as well as arthritic knee pain [68, 72, 73]. Furthermore, topical diclofenac has been shown to be effective in reducing myofascial pain, however, with no effect on the myofascial trigger point pain threshold [74]. Topical NSAIDs have been shown to have equal efficacy as oral NSAIDs, yet various studies have shown topical diclofenac to reduce pain within 2–3 days of treatment [72, 75–77].

Neuropathic pain has been shown to respond to topical agents. For example, topical lidocaine, when used in post-herpetic neuralgia (PHN), has been associated with improved quality of life, improvement of pain and allodynia [78]. Moreover, when compared with oral pregabalin, response rates were higher in patients with either PHN or diabetic neuropathy. The same studies also showed a lower rate of adverse events and improved quality of life [77, 79, 80]. Topical capsaicin cream has also been studied to reduce neuropathic pain; nonetheless, application of this cream has been associated with a burning sensation in up to 81% of patients [81]. Randomized controlled studies of high concentration topical capsaicin revealed significant pain relief in patients with PHN with relief lasting up to 12 weeks [77, 82, 83].

Topical opioids have not been shown to significantly reduce pain. For example, a randomized controlled trial comparing the use of topical morphine sulfate versus traditional Jelonet dressings in burn patients revealed increased need of rescue analgesia and higher pain scores in the topical morphine group [84]. Another study revealed no significant reduction in pain with patients with skin ulcers when topical morphine was compared to placebo [85]. However, in patients with mucositis undergoing chemoradiotherapy for head and neck cancer, oral morphine mouthwash has been shown to significantly reduce pain and reduce length of functional impairment [86]

In summary, topical analgesics may provide additional analgesia in patients who may not be able to tolerate the adverse effects of systemic analgesics. Those with PHN may benefit from topical lidocaine when amitriptyline fails to provide relief. Those with peptic ulcer disease may benefit from topical NSAIDs to treat arthritis, as oral NSAIDs may worsen their condition. By contrast, topical opioids have not been shown to provide significant relief in burns or skin conditions, limiting their role in the ED.

3.3. Peripheral nerve blocks

There are two types of nerve blocks: single injection and continuous nerve blocks.

Single-injection nerve blocks are one-time injections of local anesthetic adjacent to the nerve or plexus for anesthesia and/or analgesia and are most commonly used in the ED. Continuous infusion nerve blocks involve the placement of catheter adjacent to the peripheral nerve or plexus. These are useful in patients who are expected to have prolonged need for analgesia. The effectiveness and duration of the block depend upon the pharmacology of the analgesic/anesthetic agent used, the dose, and the concentration.

Peripheral nerve blocks are important tools for pain management in the ED and have been shown to significantly reduce pain. Analgesia from peripheral nerve blocks can be reached more quickly than intravenous narcotics and often with more efficacy and less rescue analgesics. A randomized controlled trial compared the use of femoral nerve blocks versus intravenous narcotics in femoral fractures and found lower pain scores within 90 minutes in the femoral nerve block group. The incidence of infections was the same in both groups, and there were no reports of paresthesias [87]. In fact, the total amount of morphine required to produce adequate analgesia was up to three times higher in intravenous narcotics group than in patients with a peripheral nerve block [88].

The benefits of peripheral nerve blocks have not only been seen in femoral fractures but also in other traumatic injuries such as hand lacerations, upper extremity fractures, and dislocations. For reduction of forearm fractures, studies have shown that children have less distress and pain when a brachial plexus block was performed versus procedural sedation [89]. Furthermore, length of stay in the ED was also significantly reduced when brachial plexus block was performed with length of stay being reduced almost 3 hours [90]. Similarly, patients with shoulder dislocation that underwent a brachial plexus block also showed reduction in ED length of stay, without any increased adverse events or reduction in patient satisfaction [91].

One of the most concerning complications of peripheral nerve blocks is nerve damage. In a peripheral nerve block, the goal is to position the local anesthetic around the nerve and not "into" the nerve. One should avoid intra-neural injection that may cause direct trauma or toxicity to the nerve. The incidence of nerve damage in the days following the block (including temporary paresthesias) ranges from 0.5 to 15% [92, 93]. However, in significant nerve damage resulting in peripheral neuropathy or symptoms lasting longer than 6 months, incidence was reported to be less than 0.1% in a prospective study [92, 94]. Most complications of nerve damage are transient, with most patients recovering by 3 weeks. Localized infection has been noted to be rare, with 3% of peripheral nerve catheters in anesthesia studies showing signs of infection or abscess formation [95]. On the contrary, vascular puncture is not uncommon, and incidences of up to 5.7% and 6.6% have been noted when investigators placed femoral or sciatic nerve peripheral catheters [92, 96]. Systemic toxicity, such as cardiac arrest, was found to be rare, with all cases of cardiac arrest noted to be in central spinal anesthesia. Additionally, seizures were noted in 6 out of 50,223 cases [94].

Ultrasound and nerve stimulator techniques have been shown to reduce the complications from peripheral nerve blocks. One study investigating the use of ultrasound or electrical stimulation in the placement of a brachial plexus peripheral nerve catheter resulted not only in decreased time performing the procedure but also no vascular punctures in the ultrasound-guided group [97]. Furthermore, a Cochrane systematic review also confirmed faster procedure times and reduced local anesthetic volume and improved quality of nerve block [98].

Emergency physicians are adept at using ultrasound in central line placement, as well as in other diagnostic procedures, such as in FAST abdominal examinations, in trauma patients. Emergency physicians can be trained in ultrasound-guided peripheral nerve blocks as well. Ultrasound imaging permits direct visualization of needle location relative to target nerves, blood vessels, and related structures, as well as observation of the local anesthetic during and after the injection. A prospective observational study trained emergency physicians in the use of ultrasound guided peripheral nerve blocks in patients with traumatic limb emergencies and found that trained physicians were able to perform the ultrasound-guided nerve blocks in about 9 minutes with no complications and no need of rescue procedural sedation [99].

Prior to the decision to perform a peripheral nerve block, a careful medical history should be obtained including allergies, use of anticoagulants, preexisting nerve damage, active infections at the site, and ability to cooperate with the procedures. During the placement of peripheral nerve bocks, patients should be carefully monitored. It is important to assess for preexisting sensory or motor deficits in the distribution of the block. A patient with neurologic deficits prior to the nerve block may be at higher risk for developing new neurologic deficits following a nerve block than a patient without preexisting deficits. A brief overview of the femoral and brachial plexus peripheral nerve will be explained in the section below.

3.4. Femoral nerve block

The femoral nerve block is used to anesthetize the hip, anterior thigh, and knee. This nerve passes beneath the inguinal ligament and travels lateral to the femoral artery within the femoral triangle (**Figure 1**) [100]. The fascia iliaca separates the femoral nerve from the femoral vascular bundle [101]. The patient is initially positioned in a supine position. The affected extremity is then externally rotated and abducted. With the probe marker to the patient's right, a linear probe is then placed at the inguinal crease parallel to the inguinal ligament, the femoral nerve will then be visualized (it may appear as a hyper echoic, honeycombed structure). Medially, the femoral artery and then the femoral vein will be present. The iliopsoas muscle will be present posteriorly and the fascia lata superiorly (**Figure 2**) [101, 102].

http://dx.doi.org/10.5772/62861

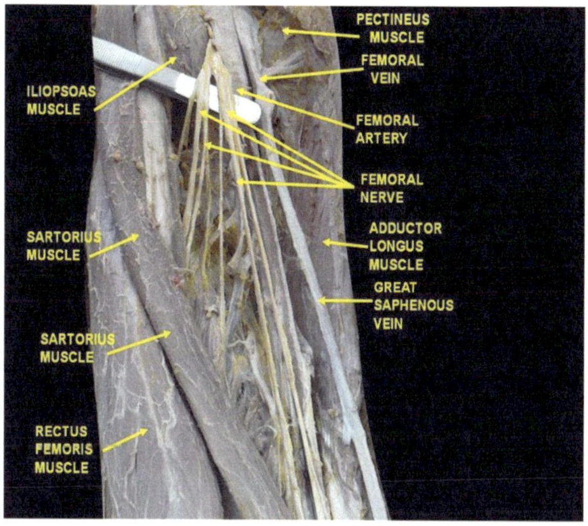

Figure 1. Femoral triangle.

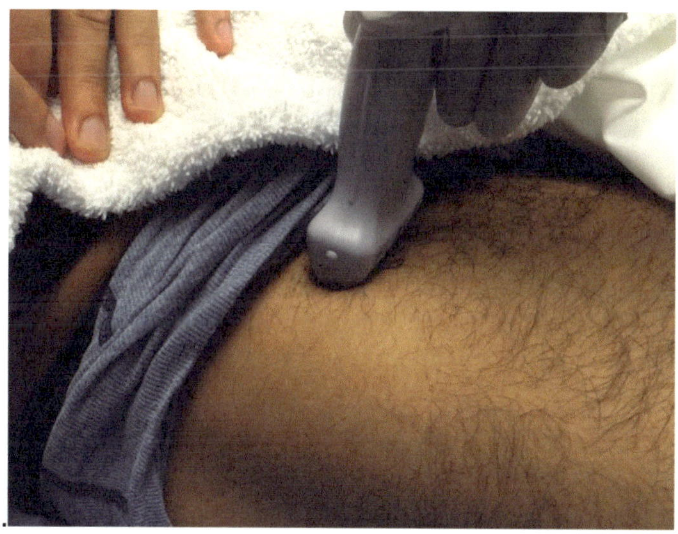

Figure 2. Placement of the ultrasound linear probe for the femoral nerve block. The patient is laid in a supine position with the affected extremity externally rotated and abducted. The linear probe is placed in a transverse fashion inferiorly to the inguinal crease.

Once the structures and anatomical landmarks mentioned above have been identified, aseptic skin preparation is performed and anatomic structures at the block site are again identified using an ultrasound probe in a sterile plastic sheath with sterile conductive gel (**Figure 3**). The structures are once again confirmed on ultrasound and then a skin wheal is made with local anesthetic. When the optimal ultrasound view is achieved, the probe is held immobile; the block needle is then inserted at the skin on the lateral edge of the probe in-plane, aiming for the space behind the nerve. It is then advanced, with movement only when the needle tip is seen. Often a "pop" will be felt as the fascia iliaca is penetrated with the needle. Next, aspiration of the needle is done to confirm no vascular penetration. About 1–2 ml of local anesthetic is injected to visualize the placement of the needle on the ultrasound screen. The anesthetic should be seen surrounding the nerve. Once correct placement is confirmed, 10–20 ml of the selected anesthetic is injected. It may take up to 10–20 minutes to take effect [101–103].

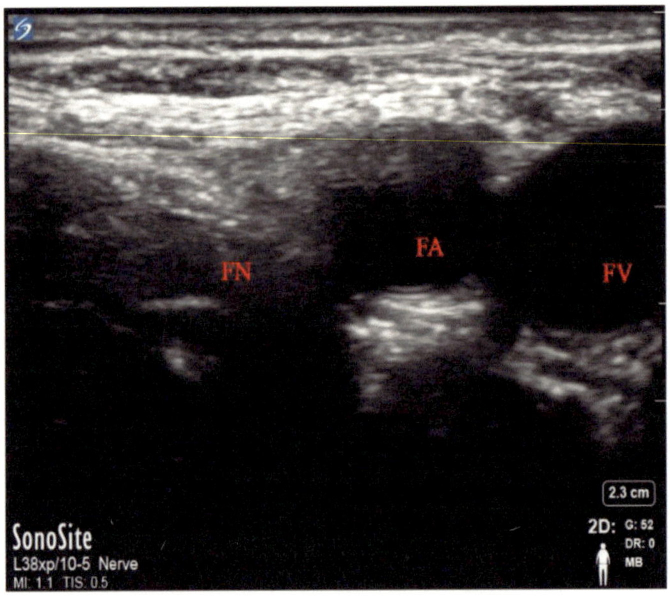

Figure 3. Ultrasound view of the femoral nerve. FA, femoral artery; FV, femoral vein; FN, femoral nerve.

3.5. Brachial plexus block

The brachial plexus block, or interscalene block, can be used to facilitate reduction of upper extremity fractures, lacerations, and even reduce shoulder dislocations. Nerve roots of C5-T1 are the initial part of the brachial plexus, forming a complex configuration before they enter the terminal nerves of the arm (**Figure 4**) [104]. The more proximal one blocks to the plexus, the more proximal the anesthesia is on the arm. Nerve roots of C5-T1 form the superior, middle, and inferior trunks of the plexus at the level of the cricoid cartilage. At this location, the plexus is found superior and posterior to the subclavian artery, with the dome of the lung located anteromedial to the inferior trunk. The interscalene space is the grove between the anterior and middle scalene muscles. This is where one will find the structures mentioned above. However, since the inferior trunk is often not included in this block, one cannot use this procedure for injuries below the elbow [105].

http://dx.doi.org/10.5772/62861

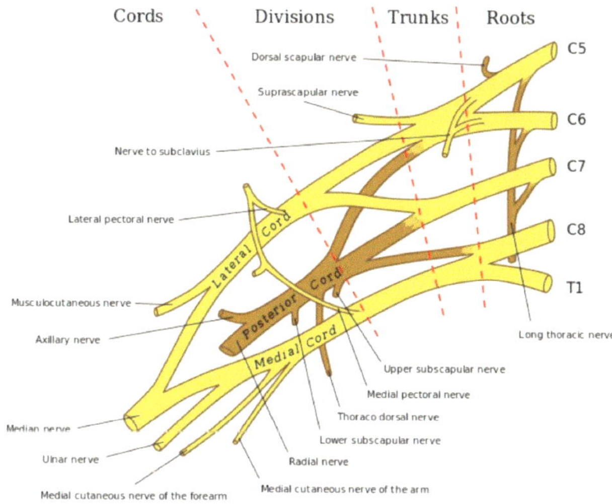

Figure 4. Brachial plexus.

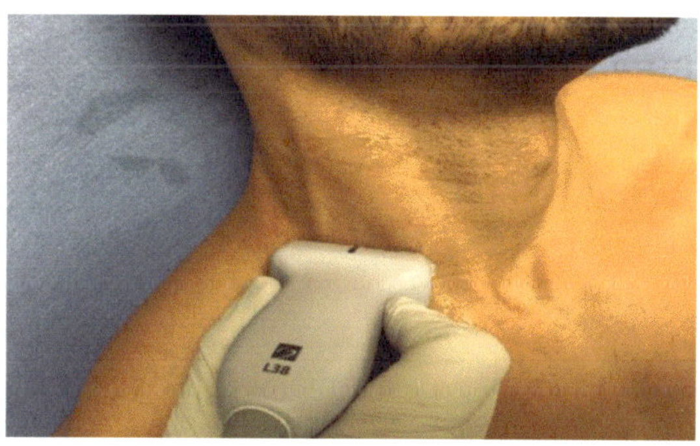

Figure 5. Placement of the ultrasound linear probe for the interscalene brachial plexus block. The patient is laid in a supine position with head turned away. The probe is then placed in a transverse fashion and used to identify the sternocleidomastoid muscle first. Next, one then sweeps posterior laterally to bring into view the interscalene groove.

The patient is initially positioned supine with the head turned 45 degrees to the contralateral side. With a linear probe, one first identifies the sternocleidomastoid muscle (SCM), which is located anteriorly to the carotid artery and internal jugular vein. One then sweeps posterior laterally bringing into view the middle scalene muscle and anterior scalene muscles. This is where the trunks of the brachial plexus may be visualized between the anterior and middle interscalene muscles. As with peripheral nerves, these trunks may appear as hyper echoic honeycombed structures (**Figure 5**) [105, 106]. Once the structures are identified, aseptic skin preparation is performed and anatomic structures at the block site are again identified using an ultrasound probe in a sterile plastic sheath with sterile conductive gel. A skin wheal is made using local anesthetic. Then, in an in-plane approach, the block needle is inserted posterior-laterally to the probe, at an angle of 45 degrees to the skin. The needle is advanced toward the plexus, aiming toward the space between the top and middle trunks. Next, aspiration is done to check for any vascular puncture, and then placement is confirmed with movement of the trunks on injection of anesthetic. Depending on the agent used, the volume of local anesthetic is about 15–45 ml (**Figure 6**) [105, 106].

A second approach to the brachial plexus block is a supraclavicular block. To perform this block, the patient is once again laid in a supine position with the head turned away from the side being blocked. A linear probe transducer is then placed immediately superior to the clavicle at its midpoint (**Figure 7**). Tilting the probe caudally will bring into view a transverse view of the subclavian artery. Laterally to the artery, one will be able to see a collection of hypo echoic, honeycombed structures, which is the brachial plexus. Underneath these structures, the first rib is visible as a linear hyper echoic structure with lung underneath (**Figure 8**) [107, 108]. After the correct anatomy is identified, the skin is prepped in a sterile manner, and using a sterile probe cover, this area is once again identified. A 27-gauge needle is then used to inject the skin with 1–2 ml of local anesthetic just lateral to the probe. The block needle, 22-gauge, is then advanced in an in-plane approach toward the brachial plexus from a lateral to medial direction. At times one may feel a "pop" once the brachial sheath has been penetrated. One then aspirates to confirm non-vascular penetration and injects 1–2 ml of anesthetic to view the brachial plexus. Next, one then injects about 20–25 ml of anesthetic, until adequate spread is seen surrounding the brachial plexus [107].

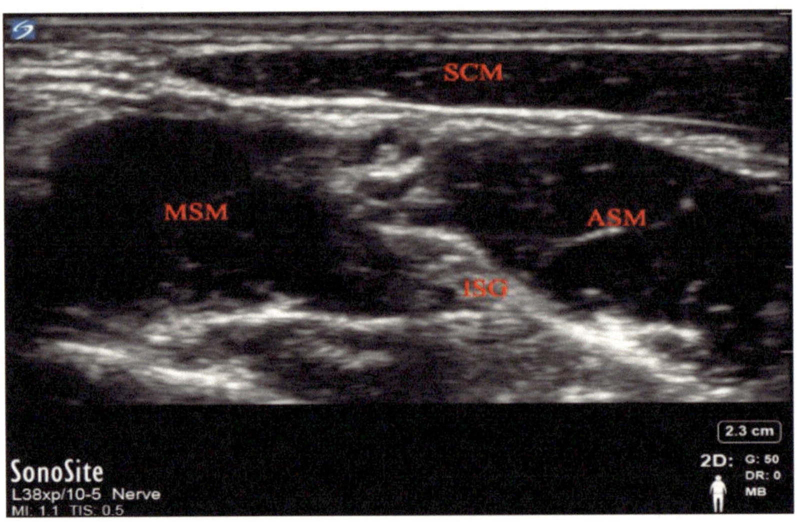

Figure 6. Interscalene view of the brachial plexus. ISG, interscalene groove with the brachial plexus present; SCM, sternocleidomastoid muscle; ASM, anterior scalene muscle; MSM, middle scalene muscle.

http://dx.doi.org/10.5772/62861

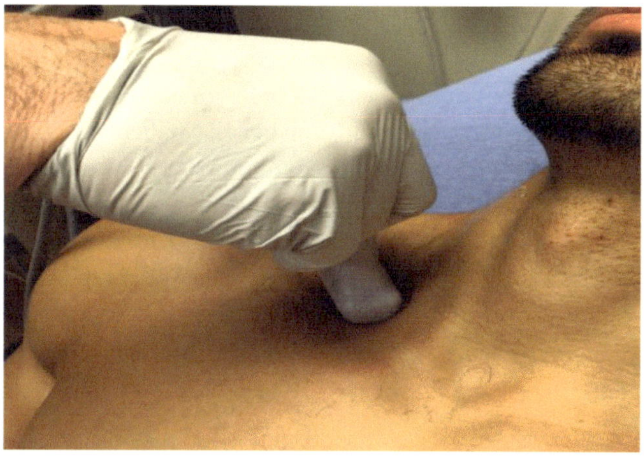

Figure 7. Placement of the ultrasound linear probe for the supraclavicular brachial plexus block. The patient is placed in a supine position or slightly seated position. The linear probe is then placed immediately superior to the clavicle at its midpoint. Tilting the probe caudally will bring into view the subclavian artery with the brachial plexus seen lateral to it, and the first rib and lung underneath.

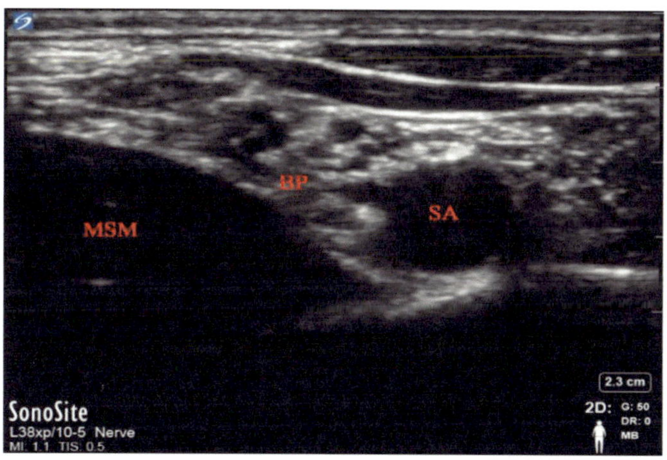

Figure 8. Supraclavicular view of the brachial plexus. SA, subclavian artery; BP, brachial plexus; MSM, middle scalene muscle.

Peripheral nerve blocks are a valuable asset to the emergency physician trained in these procedures. These procedures reduce pain quicker than intravenous narcotics, decrease the amount of sedation needed, and decrease ED length of stays. Peripheral nerve blocks may offer an alternative to avoid respiratory and cardiovascular depression encountered with procedural sedation or intravenous narcotics.

4. Conclusion

Pain is the most common presenting complaint to the emergency room. Appropriate treatment affects not only patient satisfaction and well-being but also patient outcomes. The choice of an appropriate initial therapeutic strategy is dependent upon an accurate evaluation of the cause of the pain and the type of pain syndrome. Effective management of acute pain in the ED requires a systematic approach. First, an accurate assessment of the patient's pain should involve the use of validated pain scales. Second, suitable analgesics given in an acceptable time frame are essential in the diagnosis and treatment. This should include proper monitoring for adverse side effects. Third, pain should be reassessed and documented regularly to determine the effect of treatment.

Author details

Ivan Samcam MD and Linda Papa MD, MSc*

*Address all correspondence to: lpstat@aol.com

Orlando Regional Medical Center, Orlando, FL, USA

References

[1] McCaig LF, Stussman BJ. National Hospital Ambulatory Medical Care Survey: 1996 Emergency Department Summary. Advance Data from Vital and Health Statistics. National Center for Health Statistics. 1997;293. http://www.cdc.gov/nchs/data/ad/ad293.pdf

[2] CDC. Emergency Department Visits 2015 [cited 12/28/2015]. Available from: http://www.cdc.gov/nchs/fastats/emergency-department.htm.

[3] Pitts S, Niska RW, Xu J, Burt C. National Hospital Ambulatory Medical Care Survey: 2006 Emergency Department Summary. National Health Statistics Report. 2008;7:1–39.

[4] Motov SM, Khan AN. Problems and barriers of pain management in the emergency department: are we ever going to get better? J Pain Res. 2009;2:5–11.

[5] Wilson J, Pendleton J. Oligoanalgesia in the emergency department. Am J Emer Med. 1989;7(6):620–3.

[6] Lewis L, Lasater L, Brooks C. Are emergency physicians too stingy with analgesics? South Med J. 1994;87:7–9.

[7] Blank F, Mader T, Wolfe J, Keyes M, Kirschner R, Provost D. Adequacy of pain assessment and pain relief and correlation of patient satisfaction in 68 ED fast-track patients. J Emerg Nurs. 2001;27:327–34.

[8] Todd K, Ducharme J, Choiniere M, Group PS. Pain in the emergency department: results of the pain and emergency medicine (PEMI) multicenter study. J Pain. 2007;8:460–6.

[9] Fosnocht D, Heaps N, Swanson E. Patient expectations for pain relief in the ED. Am J Emerg Med. 2004;22:286–8.

[10] Downey LVA, Zun LS. Pain management in the emergency department and its relationship to patient satisfaction. J Emerg Trauma Shock. 2010;3(4):326–30.

[11] Kim M, Strait R, Sato T, Hennes H. A randomized clinical trial of analgesia in children with acute abdominal pain. Acad Emerg Med. 2002;9:281–7.

[12] Yong Y, Jia-yong C, Hao G, Yi Z, Dao-Ming L, Dong Z, et al. Relief of abdominal pain by morphine without altering physical signs in acute appendicitis. Chin Med J. 2010;123(2):142–5.

[13] Poonai N, Paskar D, Konrad S-L, Rieder M, Joubert G, Lim R, et al. Opioid analgesia for acute abdominal pain in children: a systematic review and meta-analysis. Acad Emerg Med. 2014;21(11):1185–992.

[14] CDC. Opioid Painkiller Prescribing 2014 [cited 01/20/2016]. Available from: http://www.cdc.gov/vitalsigns/opioid-prescribing/.

[15] Birnbaum H, White A, Schiller M. Societal costs of prescription opioid abuse, dependence and misuse in the United States. Pain Med. 2011;12(4):657–67.

[16] Wilsey B, Fishman SM, Tsodikov A, Ogden BS, Symreg I, Ernst A. Psychological comorbidities predicting prescription opioid abuse among patients in chronic pain presenting to the emergency department. Pain Med. 2008;9(8):1107–17.

[17] Edlund M, Steffick D, Hudson T, Harris K, Sullivan M. Risk factors for clinically recognized opioid abuse and dependence among veterans using opioids for chronic non-cancer pain. Pain. 2007;129(3):355–62.

[18] Silka PA, Mendel MR, Moreno G, Merrill L, Geiderman JM. Pain scores improve analgesic administration patterns for trauma patients in the emergency department. Acad Emerg Med. 2008;11(3):264–70.

[19] Pines JM, Hollander JE. Emergency department crowding is associated with poor care for patients with severe pain. Ann Emerg Med. 2007;51(1):1–5.

[20] Miner JR, Burton J. Pain Management. In: Marx JA, Hockberger RS, Walls RM, Biros MH, editors. Rosen's Emergency Medicine 1. 8th ed. Philadelphia, PA: Elsevier Saunders; 2014. pp. 31–49.

[21] Rosenquist RW, Vrooman B. Chronic Pain Management. In: Butterworth JF, Mackey DC, Wasnick JD, editors. Morgan and MIkhail's Clinical Anesthesiology. Regional Anesthesia and Pain Management. New York, NY: McGraw-Hill Companies; 2013.

[22] Woolf CJ, Doubell TP. The pathophysiology of chronic pain—increased sensitivity to low threshold Aβ-fibre inputs. Curr Opin Neurobiol. 1994;4(4):525–34.

[23] Rexed B. The cytoarchitecture organization of the spinal cord in the cat. J Comp Neurol. 1952;96(3):414–95.

[24] Schoenen, J.,Grant G. Spinal Cord: connections. In Paxinos G, Mai JK, editors. The Human Nervous System. 2 ed. San Diego, 2004. Elsevier Academic Press, page 236.

[25] Holstege G. Direct and indirect pathways to lamina 1 in the medulla oblongata and spinal cord of the cat. Prog Brain Res. 1988;77:47–94.

[26] Behbehani MM. Functional characteristics of the midbrain periaqueductal gray. Prog Neurobiol. 1995;46:575–605.

[27] Reynolds DV. Surgery in the rat during electrical analgesia by focal brain stimulation. Science. 1969;164:444–5.

[28] Onghena P, Van Houdenhove B. Antidepressant-induced analgesia in chronic non-malignant pain: a meta-analysis of 39 placebo-controlled studies. Pain. 1992;49:205–19.

[29] Thomas S. Management of Pain in the Emergency Department. ISRN Emergency Medicine. 2013;2013:19.

[30] Patanwala AE, Edwards CJ, Stolz L, Amini R, Desai A, Stolz U. Should morphine dosing be weight based for analgesia in the emergency department? J Opioid Manag. 2012;8:51–5.

[31] Bliur P, Kenny M, Gallagher E. Intravenous morphine at 0.1 mg/kg is not effective for controlling severe acute pain in the majority of patients. Ann Emerg Med. 2005;46(4): 362–7.

[32] Farsi D, Movahedi M, Hafezimpghadam P, Abbasi S, Shahlaee A, Rahimi-Movaghar V. Acute pain management with intravenous 0.10 mg/kg vs. 0.15 mg/kg morphine sulfate in limb traumatized patients: a randomized double-blinded placebo-controlled trial. Ulus Tarvma Acil Cerr Derg. 2013;19(5):398–405.

[33] Puymirat E, Lamhaut L, Bonnet N, Aissaoui N, Henry P, Cayla G, et al. Correlates of pre-hospital morphine use in ST-elevation myocardial infarction patients and its association with in-hospital outcomes and long-term mortality: the FAST-MI (French Registry of Acute ST-elevation and non-ST-elevation Myocardial Infarction) programme. Eur Heart J. 2015;10:1–9.

[34] Citron ML, Johnston-Early A, Fossieck B, Krasnow SH, Franklin R, Spagnolo S, et al. Safety and efficacy of continuous intravenous morphine for severe cancer pain. Am J Med. 1984;77:199–204.

[35] O'Connor A, Lan V, Quil T. Underdosing of morphine in comparison with other parenteral opioids in ancute hospital. A quality of care challenge. Pain Med. 2006;7:299–307.

[36] DiGiusto M, Tarun B, David M, Derek F, Megan J, Joseph D. Patient-controlled analgesia in the pediatric population: morphine versus hydromorphone. J Pain Res. 2014;7:471–5.

[37] Chang A, Bijur P, Meyer R, Kenny M, Solorzano C, Gallagher E. Safety and efficacy of hydromorphone as an analgesic alternative to morphine in acute pain: a randomized clinical trial. Ann Emerg Med. 2006;48(2):164–72.

[38] Thomas SH, Benevelli W, Brown D, Wedel SK. Safety of fentanyl for analgesia in adults undergoing air medical transport from trauma scenes. Air Med J. 1996;15(2):57–9.

[39] Jaffe TB, Ramsey FM. Attenuation of fentanyl-induced truncal rigidity. Anesthesiology. 1983;58:562–4.

[40] Coruh B, Tonelli MR, Park DR. Fentanyl-induced chest wall rigidity. Chest. 2013;144(3):1083–4.

[41] Scwab JM, Schluesener HJ, Laufer S. COX-3: just another COX or the solitary elusive target of paracetamol? Lancet. 2003;361:981–2.

[42] Towheed TE, Hochberg MC, Judd MG, Wells G. Acetaminophen for osteoarthritis. The Cochrane Database of Systematic Reviews 2003, Issue 1. Art. No.: CD004257. DOI: 10.1002/14651858.CD004257.Full

[43] Bannuru RR, Schmid CH, Kent DM, Vaysbrot EE, Wong JB, McAlindon TE. Comparative effectiveness of pharmacologic interventions for knee osteoarthritis: a systematic review and network meta-analysis. Ann Intern Med. 2015;162(1):46–54.

[44] Shen H, Sprott H, Aeschillmann A, Gay RE, Michel BA, Gay S. Analgesic action of acetaminophen in symptomatic osteoarthritis of the knee. Oxford. 2006;45:765–70.

[45] Craig M, Jeavons R, Probert J, Benger J. Randomised comparison of intravenous paracetamol and intravenous morphine for acute traumatic limb pain in the emergency department. Emerg Med J. 2012;29(1):37–9.

[46] Esmailian M, Moshiri R, Majid Z. Comparison of the analgesic effect of intravenous acetaminophen and morphine sulfate in rib fracture: a randomized double-blind clinical trial. Emergency. 2015;3(3):99–102.

[47] Sinatra RS, Jahr JS, Reynolds L, Groudine S, Royal M, Breitmeyer JB, et al. Intravenous acetaminophen for pain after major orthopedic surgery: an expanded analysis. Pain Pract. 2011;12(5):357–65.

[48] Wininger SJ, Miller H, Minkowitz HS, Royal M, Ang R, Breitmeyer JB, et al. A randomized, double-blind, placebo-controlled, multicenter, repeat-dose study of two intrave-

nous acetaminophen dosing regimens for the treatment of pain after abdominal laparoscopic surgery. Clin Ther. 2010;32(14):2348–69.

[49] Macario A, Royal M. A literature review of randomized clinical trials of intravenous acetaminophen (paracetamol) for acute postoperative pain. Pain Pract. 2010;11(3):290–6.

[50] Mernis D, Mehmet TI, Guksum K, Sezer A, Sut N. Intravenous paracetamol reduced the use of opioids, extubation time, and opioid-related adverse effects after major surgery in intensive care unit. J Crit Care. 2010;25(3):458–62.

[51] Golzari SE, Soleimanpour H, Rahmani F, et al. Therapeutic Approaches for Renal Colic in the Emergency Department: A Review Article. Anesthesiology and Pain Medicine. 2014;4(1):e16222. doi:10.5812/aapm.16222.

[52] Lafrance JP, Miller DR. Selective and non-selective non-steroidal anti-inflammatory drugs and the risk of acute kidney injury. Pharmacoepidemiol Drug Saf. 2009;10:923–31.

[53] Masso Gonzalex EL, Patrignani P, Taconelli S, Garcia Rodriguez LA. Variability among nonsteroidal antiinflammatory drugs in risk of upper gastrointestinal bleeding. Arthritis Rheum. 2010;62(6):1592–601.

[54] Fitzgerald G. Coxibs and cardiovascular disease. New Engl J Med. 2004;351:1709–11.

[55] Solomon DH, Schneeweiss S, Glynn RJ, Kiyota Y, Levin R, Mogun H, et al. Relationship between selective cyclooxygenase-2 inhibitors and acute myocardial infarction in older adults. Circulation. 2004;109:2068–73.

[56] Ray WA, Stein CM, Daugherty JR, Hall K, Arbogast PG, Grfiffin MR. COX-2 selective non-steroidal anti-inflammatory drugs and increased risk of serious coronary heart disease. Lancet. 2002;360:1071–3.

[57] Rios A, Vargas-Robles H, Gamez-Mendez AM, Escalante B. Cyclooxygenase-2 and kidney failure. Prostag Oth Lipid Med. 2012;98:86–90.

[58] Green T, Gonzalez AA, Mitchell KD, Navar LG. The complex interplay between cyclooxygenase-2 ans angiotensin II in regulating kidney function. Curr Opin Nephrol Hy. 2012;21:7–14.

[59] Turturro MA, Paris PM, Seaberg DC. Intramuscular ketorolac versus oral ibuprofen in acute musculoskeletal pain. Ann Emerg Med. 1995;26(2):117–20.

[60] Wright JM, Price SD, Watson WA. NSAID use and efficacy in the emergency department: single doses oral ibuprofen versus intramuscular ketorolac. Ann Pharmacother. 1994;28(3):309–12.

[61] Jelinek G. Ketorolac versus morphine for severe pain. BMJ. 2000;321(7271):1236–7.

[62] Safdar B, Degutis LC, Landry K, Vedere SR, Moscovitz HC, D'Onofrio G. Intravenous morphine versus ketorolac is superior to either drug alone for treatment of acute renal colic. Ann Emerg Med. 2006;48(2):173–81.

[63] van Tulder MW, Scholten RJ, Koes BW, Deyo RA. Non-steroidal anti-inflammatory drugs for low back pain. Cochrane Database Syst Rev. 2000;25(19):2501–13.

[64] Friedman BW, Dym AA, Davitt M, Holden L, Solorzano C, Esses D, et al. Naproxen with cyclobenzaprine, oxycodone/acetaminophen, or placebo for treating low back pain: a randomized clinical trial. JAMA. 2015;314(15):1572–80.

[65] van Tulder MW, Touray T, Furlan AD, Solway S, Bouter LM, Group CBR. Muscle relaxants for nonspecific low back pain: a systematic review within the framework of the cochrane collaboration. Spine. 2003;28(17):1978–92.

[66] Peloso PMJ, Gross A, Haines T, Trinh K, Goldsmith CH, Burnie SJ, Cervical Overview Group. Medicinal and injection therapies for mechanical neck disorders. Cochrane Database of Systematic Reviews 2007, Issue 3. Art. No.: CD000319. DOI: 10.1002/14651858.CD000319.pub4.

[67] Khwaja SM, Minnerop M, Singer AJ. Comparison of ibuprofen, cyclobenzaprine, or both in patients with acute cervical strain: a randomized controlled trial. Can J Emerg Med. 2010;12(1):39–44.

[68] Tiso RL, Tong-Ngork S, Fredlund KL. Oral versus topical ibuprofen for chronic knee pain: a prospective randomized pilot study. Pain Physician. 2010;13(5):457–67.

[69] Heyneman CA, Lawless-Liday C, Wall GC. Oral versus topical NSAIDs in rheumatic diseases: a comparison. Drugs. 2000;60(3):555–74.

[70] Paice JA, Von Roerin JH, Hudgins JC, Luong L, Krejcie TC, Avram MJ. Morphine bioavailability from a topical gel formulation in volunteers. J Pain Symptom Manage. 2008;35(3):314–20.

[71] Jorge LL, Feres CC, Teles VE. Topical preparations for pain relief: efficacy and patient adherence. J Pain Res. 2011;4:11–24.

[72] Constantino C, Kwarecki J, Samokhin AV, Mautone G, Rovati S. Diclofenac epolamine plus heparin plaster versus diclofenac epolamine plaster in mild to moderate ankle sprain, a randomized double blind, parallel-group, placebo-controlled, multi-centre, phase III trial. Clin Drug Invest. 2011;31(1):15–26.

[73] Baer PA, Thomas LM, Shainhouse Z. Treatment of osteoarthritis of the knee with a topical diclofenac solution, a randomised controlled 6-week trial. BMC Musculoskeletal Disord. 2005;6:44.

[74] Hsieh LF, Hong CZ, Chern SH, Chen CC. Efficacy and side effects of diclofenac patch in treatment of patients with myofascial pain syndrome of the upper trapezius. J Pain Symptom Manage. 2010;39(1):116–25.

[75] Mueller EA, Kirch W, Reiter S. Extent and time course of pain intensity upon treatment with a topical diclofenac sodium patch versus placebo in acute traumatic injury based on validated end-point: post hoc analysis of a randomized placebo-controlled trial. Expert Opin Pharmacother. 2010;11(4):493–8.

[76] Galer BS, Rowbothan M, Perander J, Devers A, Friedman E. Topical diclofenac patch relieves minor sports injury pain: results of a multicenter controlled clinical trial. J Clin Pharmacol. 2000;19(4):287–94.

[77] Argoff CE. Topical analgesics in the management of acute and chronic pain. Mayo Clin Proc. 2013;88(2):195–205.

[78] Brider A, Bruxelle J, Rogers P, Hans G, Bosl I, Baron R. Topical 5% lidocaine (lignocaine) medicated plaster treatment for post-herptic neuralgia: results of a double-blind, placebo-controlled, multinational efficacy and safety trial. Clin Drug Invest. 2009;29(6): 393–408.

[79] Baron R, Mayoral V, Leijon G, Binder A, Steigerwald I, Serpell M. 5% Lidocaine medicated plaster versus pregabalin in post-herpetic neuralgia and diabetic polyneuropathy: an open label, non-inferiority two-stage RCT study. Curr Med Res Opin. 2009;25(7):1663–76.

[80] Baron R, Mayoral V, Leijon G, Binder A, Steigerwald I, Serpell M. Efficacy and safety of 5% lidocaine (lignocaine) medicated plaster in comparison with pregabalin in patients with post-herpetic neuralgia and diabetic polyneuropathy: interim analysis from an open-label, two-stage adaptive, randomized controlled trial. Clin Drug Invest. 2009;29(4):231–41.

[81] McCleane G. Topical application of doxepin hydrochloride, capsaicin and a combination of both produces analgesia in chronic human neuropathic pain: a randomized, double-blind, placebo-controlled study. Br J Clin Pharmacol. 2000;49(6):574–9.

[82] Backonja MM, Malan TP, Vanhove GF, Tobias JK, Group CS. NGX-4010, a high concentration capsaicin patch, for the treatment of post-herpetic neuralgia: a randomized, double-blind, controlled study with an open-label extension. Pain Med. 2010;11(4):600–8.

[83] Irving GA, Backonja MM, Dunteman E, Group N-CS. A multicenter randomized, double-blind, controlled study of NGX-4010, a high-concentration capsaicin patch, for the treatment of postherpetic neuralgia. Pain Med. 2011;12(1):99–109.

[84] Welling A. A randomised controlled trial to test the analgesic efficacy of topical morphine on minor superficial and partial thickness burns in accident and emergency departments. Emerg Med J. 2007;24:408–12.

[85] Vernassiere C, Cornet C, Trechot P, Alla F, Truchetet F, Cuny JF, et al. Study to determine the efficacy of topical morphine on painful chronic skin ulcers. J Wound Care. 2005;14(6):289–93.

[86] Cerchietti L, Navigante AH, Bonomi MR, Zaderajko MA, Menendez PR, Pogany CE, et al. Study to determine the efficacy of topical morphine on painful chronic skin ulcers. Cancer. 2002;95(10):2230–6.

[87] Mutty CE, Jensen EJ, Manka MA, Anders MJ, Bone LB. Femoral nerve block for diaphyseal and distal femoral fractures in the emergency department. J Bone Joint Surg Am. 2007;89:12.

[88] Fletcher A, Rigby A, Heyes F. Three-in-one femoral nerve block as analgesia for fractured neck of femur in the emergency department: a randomized, controlled trial. Ann Emerg Med. 2003;41(2):227–33.

[89] Kriwanek K, Wan J, Beaty J, Pershad J. Axillary block for analgesia during manipulation of forearm fractures in the pediatric emergency department: a prospective randomized comparative trial. J Pediatr Orthop. 2006;26(6):737–40.

[90] Stone MB, Wang R, Price DD. Ultrasound-guided supraclavicular brachial plexus nerve block vs procedural sedation for the treatment of upper extremity emergencies. Am J Emerg Med. 2008;26(6):706–10.

[91] Blaivas M, Adhikari S, Liander L. A prospective comparison of procedural sedation and ultrasound-guided interscalene nerve block for shoulder reduction in the emergency department. Acad Emerg Med. 2011;18(9):922–7.

[92] Jeng CL, Torrillo TM, Rosenblatt MA. Complications of peripheral nerve blocks. Br J Anaesth. 2010;105:i97–i107.

[93] Liguori GA. Complications of regional anesthesia: nerve injury and peripheral neural blockade. J Neurosurg Anesthesiol. 2004;16(1):84–6.

[94] Auroy Y, Benhamou D, Bargues L, Ecoffey C, Falissard B, Mercier F, et al. Major complications of regional anesthesia in France. The SOS Regional Anesthesia Hotline Service. Anesthesiology. 2002;97:1274–80.

[95] Capdevilla X, Bringuier S, Borgeat A. Infectious risk of continuous peripheral nerve blocks. Anesthesiology. 2009;110:182–8.

[96] Wiegel M, Gottschaldt U, Hennebach R, Hirshberg T, Reske A. Complications and adverse effects associated with continuous peripheral nerve blocks in orthopedic patients. Anesth and Analg. 2007;104(6):1578–82.

[97] Mariano ER, Loland VJ, Bellars RH, Sandhu NS, Bishop ML, Abrams RA, et al. Ultrasound guidance versus electrical stimulation for infraclavicular brachial plexus perineural catheter insertion. J Ultrasound Med. 2009;28:1211–8.

[98] Walker KJ, McGrattan K, Aas-Eng K, Smith AF. Ultrasound guidance for peripheral nerve blockade. Cochrane Database of Systematic Reviews 2009, Issue 4. Art. No.: CD006459. DOI: 10.1002/14651858.CD006459.pub2.

[99] Bhoi S, Sinha TP, Rodha M, Bhasin A, Ramchandani R, Galwankar S. Feasibility and safety of ultrasound-guided nerve block for management of limb injuries by emergency care physicians. J Emerg, Trauma Shock. 2012;5(1):28–32.

[100] Anatomist 90. Femoral Triangle. In: File:Slide6888.JPG, editor. Wikipedia: Creative Commons Attribution-ShareAlike License; 2015. p. Femoral Triangle.

[101] Otterness K, Vermeulen M. Practical tips: when and how to use a femoral nerve block. EM Resident Magazine [Internet] [cited 12/18/2015]; 2014.

[102] Dewitz A, Jones RA, Goldsetin JG, Stone MB. Additional Ultrasound Guided Procedures. In: Ma O, Mateer JR, Reardon RF, Joing SA, editors. Ma and Mateer's Emergency Ultrasound 3e. New York: McGraw-Hill; 2014.

[103] Bunting LV, Calvello EJB. Femoral Nerve Block, 3-in-1 Block Variation. Ultrasound Guide for Emergency Physicians [Internet] [cited 12/18/2008]; 2015.

[104] Wikipedia Contributors. Brachial Plexus. In: Plexus B, editor. 694154506 ed: Wikipedia, The Free Encyclopedia; 2015. p. Brachial Plexus.

[105] Bunting LV. Interscalene Plexus Block [cited 12/21/2015]; 2008. Available from: http://www.sonoguide.com/interscalene_plexus_block.html.

[106] Borgeat A, Blumenthal S. Intersclane Plexus Block. Textbook of Regional Anesthesia. 2007. New York. McGraw-Hill. p. 413-5.

[107] Ultrasound-Guided Supraclavicular Brachial Plexus Block 2013 [updated 09/19/2013; cited 01/22/2016]. Available from: http://www.nysora.com/techniques/3015-ultrasound-guided-supraclavicular-brachial-plexus-block.html.

[108] Leech S, Samcam I. Supraclavicular view of the brachial plexus. In: Plexus SVOTB, editor. Sonosite 2016. p. Supraclavicular View of the Brachial Plexus.

Chapter 2

The Quality of Prehospital Medical Care Provided to Children with Traumatic Injuries

Anna Rutkowska and Grażyna Skotnicka-Klonowicz

Additional information is available at the end of the chapter

http://dx.doi.org/10.5772/62858

Abstract

Injuries in children reach epidemic proportions worldwide as they are the most common cause of death among children above 1 year of age. It is a well-known fact that first aid properly administered to the child with severe bodily injuries can save his or her life. That objective was pursued through a prospective analysis of data concerning the management of children who presented with an injury to the Paediatric Emergency Medicine Teaching Department at the Maria Konopnicka University Teaching Hospital No. 4, to which they were brought by emergency medical service teams or referred by a primary care physician, physicians from other hospitals or a school nurse. The study enrolled all children (1493) aged 0–18 years who, due to an injury, presented to the Paediatric Emergency Medicine Teaching Department and had had prehospital aid administered by different healthcare entities. In the group of 489 children with an injury, in whom there were indications for the administration of analgesics, only 32.8% received analgesics, while 45.6% did not receive any. In children with an injury, there was no transport immobilisation in 18%. Among children provided with transport immobilisation, 10.2% were improperly immobilised. The management of the child with an injury in the Łódzkie region is unsatisfactory.

Keywords: children, injuries, prehospital aid, analgesia, transport immobilisation

1. Introduction

For many years now, injuries in children have invariably constituted a serious medical as well as economic and social problem worldwide, as they are the most common cause of death in children above 1 year of age. Every year hundreds or even thousands of children die due to injuries and part of them suffer the irreversible consequences of sustained injuries, which prevent them from functioning in daily life. According to the World Health Organisation

(WHO), traffic accidents (22% of all unintentional injuries in the world) and violence are among main causes of deaths of young people below 18 years of age. The WHO data of 2008 indicate that about 950,000 children and adolescents die annually as a result of injuries throughout the world. What is more, it is estimated that 90% of those children lose their lives due to random accidents [1–5]. It is worth mentioning that a large majority of random injuries occur at home or in family environment; hence, a place which should ensure safety to the child. And although world organisations have implemented various prophylactic programmes aimed at decreasing the incidence of injuries among children (parents' education, introducing the duty to transport children in car safety seats and wear helmets for head protection while doing different sports), injuries in children remain a worldwide epidemic.

1.1 Injuries in children in the European Union

Paediatric injuries constitute a serious health problem in the European Union countries. Injuries are the most commonly sustained by children >5 years of age [6–8]. That is confirmed by Austrian researchers' observations which reveal that children above 5 years of age accounted for more than 50% of children with injuries, whereas children aged 1–4 years represented 28.4% and those below 1 year of age – 14% of the study group [9]. The incidence of injuries in children in Poland is not precisely determined due to the lack of the national register of paediatric injuries. According to Okłot and colleagues [6], in the 1990s about 120,000 children and adolescents were annually hospitalised as a result of injuries, including 80,000 children aged 0–14 years. Epidemiological analyses performed in consecutive years suggest a further increase in the incidence of paediatric injuries.

Boys incur injuries much more often than girls [8–12]. There was a relationship observed between sex and causes of injuries in the group of children who sustained injuries. According to the WHO, boys more commonly than girls suffer injuries owing to traffic accidents, drownings, falls and poisonings, whereas girls more often than boys sustain injuries due to burns [1].

Children most commonly incur injuries as a result of traffic accidents, drownings, burns, falls and other causes [13].

In Europe, as in the United States, traffic accidents are the main cause of deaths among children. The study by Pearson and colleagues of Glasgow indicates that main causes of deaths in the group of studied children included traffic accidents with participation of pedestrians, followed by asphyxia, assaults, burns and falls [12].

Paediatric injuries most commonly lead to traumas to the osteoarticular system and head. As common in children are burns. Recent years' studies reveal a further rise in the number of fractures within the osteoarticular system with a simultaneous fall in the number of craniocerebral injuries [9–11].

Mortality rates from injuries among children vary considerably, from the highest in Lithuania and Latvia (21.9–22.4 per 100,000) to the lowest in Sweden and the Netherlands (5.8 per 100,000), the main cause of deaths in the group of children aged 10–19 years being random accidents [1, 2]. Although observations by Finnish researchers indicate a further increase in the number of injuries in children, they simultaneously show a decrease in the mortality rate (4.0 per 100,000 of children up to 18 years of age in 2006) [11]. In Poland, children's mortality from injuries is high and the mortality rate due to accidents among children and adolescents aged 1–14 years of age is about 13.4 [14]. Epidemiological research carried out in the European Union area revealed that adolescents >15 years of age and small children up to 4 years of age bear the highest risk of mortality from injuries [2, 6, 15, 16]. As indicated by the European report on injury prevention in children, if the EU countries achieved the mortality rate from injuries in children similar to the rates in Sweden and the Netherlands, it would allow to reduce fatal consequences of injuries by 75% [7].

1.2. Prehospital management of the child with an injury

The proper administration of aid to the child with an injury requires the knowledge of the child' anatomical and physiological differences, ability to establish contact with the injured child and his/her parents/guardians, knowledge of the proper traumatic examination and interpretation of its results, as well as having at one's disposal equipment appropriate for the child.

The general protocol of managing the child with an injury is similar to that applied in adults. Upon securing the scene of the incident and initial determination of accident circumstances, the preliminary assessment of the child's condition is performed according to the International Trauma Life Support (ITLS) quick injury examination protocol. It is recommended that the systematic quick assessment of the child with an injury be performed according to the AcBCDE protocol, which allows to recognise life-threatening conditions within a few minutes.

When approaching the child, his or her general condition is assesses based on 'the first impression', that is conscious state according to the AVPU scale, patency of airways and manner of respiration, apparent injuries or bleeding. The assessment of airways is performed along with the stabilisation of the cervical spine. If airways are obstructed or their patency is threatened with the presence of foreign bodies, blood or vomit, they should be sucked out and the patency of airways should be restored manually or using devices. The cervical spine can be stabilised manually but ultimately a cervical collar of an appropriate size and subsequently a paediatric spinal board or Pedi-Pack should be used. Before applying the collar, attention should be paid to the widening of jugular veins, position of the trachea and possible wounds to the neck. When assessing the child's breathing, the respiratory rate and volume, the presence of respiratory effort and cyanosis should be checked. In the case of any respiratory difficulty, passive oxygen therapy or ventilation using a bag valve mask with a reservoir filled with pure oxygen are necessary. If tension pneumothorax is recognised, it should be decompressed as quickly as possible by puncturing the second intercostal space in the mid-clavicular line. All open chest wounds should be protected with a seal dressing [17].

When assessing the circulatory system function in the child, the first step is to secure possible external bleeding with a pressure dressing. It should be kept in mind that in the small child compensatory mechanisms allow to maintain normal systemic blood pressure in the event of loss of even up to 25% of circulating blood volume. Tachycardia and hypokinetic pulse in the child are the most definite signs of developing shock. Decreased arterial blood pressure is a late sign. When hypovolemic shock is recognised, it is essential to use intravenous fluids in order to compensate for lost blood volume by administering fluids in boluses (initial bolus is 20 ml/kg of body weight of isotonic crystalloids). In children with decompensated circulatory failure, when intravenous access is difficult to provide, intraosseous access should be considered (if attempts at providing intravenous access last more than 1 min) [6, 17–19].

The neurological assessment of the child includes the assessment of pupil widths and the evaluation of conscious state according to the Glasgow Coma Scale.

Upon performing the above actions, the next step is the quick injury examination (ITLS) of the child, paying attention to bleedings, fractures or other signs proving the sustained injury. According to standards, ITLS examination is performed from the head to feet, commencing from head and neck examination, subsequently examining the chest, abdomen, pelvis, upper and lower extremities. The child's back and buttocks are examined while transferring the child onto the board [6, 18, 19].

Prehospital aid in the case of the child with burns always consists in isolating the child from the burning agent (through undressing, removing wet or burnt clothes) with the simultaneous assessment of the child's basic vital functions. Thereafter, the extensiveness and depth of the burn wound is assessed along with its simultaneous cooling (using wet compresses). After a dozen or so minutes of cooling, the burn wound should be provided with sterile or hydrogel dressing. It is important to protect the child from hypothermia (covering with a blanket) and commence pain and shock-controlling management [20, 21].

In turn, various kinds of equipment are used to immobilise injuries to upper or lower extremities in children. The most commonly used splints are as follows: Kramer's, Sam Splint, vacuum splints. In a suspected extremity fracture, immobilisation is vital as it fulfils the following functions: analgesic, anti-inflammatory and anti-oedematous and protects against the further displacement of fragments and damage to soft tissues. In order for immobilisation to perform the above-mentioned functions, it has to be properly applied. Transport immobilisation should be well adjusted to the child's size and properly secured with bandage. It should cover the injured extremity to an appropriate extent (according to Pott's principle) [22].

Pain is always a consequence of an injury and its intensity depends on the extensiveness, severity and location of the injury. Increasing pain may lead to pain shock; hence, pain management is among the most crucial actions when administering aid to the child with an injury. Pain management is carried out non-pharmacologically, for example cooling the injured site or immobilisation of fractures, or pharmacologically.

In the case of mild pain, analgesic medicines should be administered as follows: ibuprofen 10 mg/kg of body weight every 6–8 h or paracetamol 10–15 mg/kg of body weight every 4–6 h orally or *per rectum*; maximum dose is 60 mg/kg of body weight/day. When pain is severe and IV access has been provided, analgesics ought to be administered intravenously: morphine 0.1–0.2 mg/kg of body weight or petydyna 1 mg/kg of body weight, fentanyl 1–5 mg/kg of body weight or metamizole 0.1 ml/kg of body weight [23, 24].

http://dx.doi.org/10.5772/62858

2. Assessment of medical services provided to the child with an injury

The quality of prehospital medical aid administered to the child with an injury radically affects his or her further prognosis. Nevertheless, our own observations and literature data indicate many irregularities in procedures in the prehospital period. The irregularities most commonly concern the manner of transport immobilisation, lack of IV access provision, pain management in children with burns or injuries of the osteoarticular system [25–27].

Multicentre studies assessing prehospital pain management in the child with an injury revealed that the percentage of injured children who did not undergo pain management by emergency medical service teams ranged from 22 to 70% [28, 29].

The American Academy of Pediatrics together with the American Pain Society report that main barriers to administering analgesics in children include as follows: the myth that newborns and infants feel milder pain, lack of appropriate assessment of the presence of pain, lack of knowledge of pain management and fear of side effects of analgesia including, in particular, respiratory system depression [23].

Along with studies indicating the abandonment of pain management in children with an injury, there are also isolated reports of irregularities in fracture immobilisation in children [30].

Although mistakes and oversights in the prehospital management of the child with an injury are the subject of deliberations, especially related to emergency medical service teams, the literature offers no evaluation of that management carried out by other healthcare entities.

Therefore, based on their own experience, the authors of the present study have undertaken the task of assessing the (prehospital) management of the child with an injury by different healthcare entities taking into account the manner of wound and burn dressing in children, the manner of management of fractures and dislocations within the osteoarticular system, the provision of intravenous access and pain management.

The study enrolled 1493 out of 7146 children aged 0–18 years who due to an injury presented to the Department of Paediatric Emergency Medicine (Hospital Emergency Department) at Maria Konopnicka Memorial University Teaching Hospital No. 4 from 1 May 2009 to 30 April 2010 and had received prehospital aid provided by emergency medical service teams (EMST), primary care (PC) physicians, hospital emergency departments for adults in the Łódzkie region and school nurses (**Figure 1**).

It was a prospective study which, in each child with an injury, along with demographic data, investigated information concerning: the cause, circumstances and site of the wound, entity administering medical aid, assessment of pain management, regularity of transport immobilisation, assessment of local wound and burn dressing, and assessment of medical records transferred to the Department with the child. The study used a child with injury card developed for the purposes of the study, which allowed to perform the above assessments in a uniform manner. The child with injury card was worked out based on the literature on the aetiology of paediatric injuries [26, 31, 32].

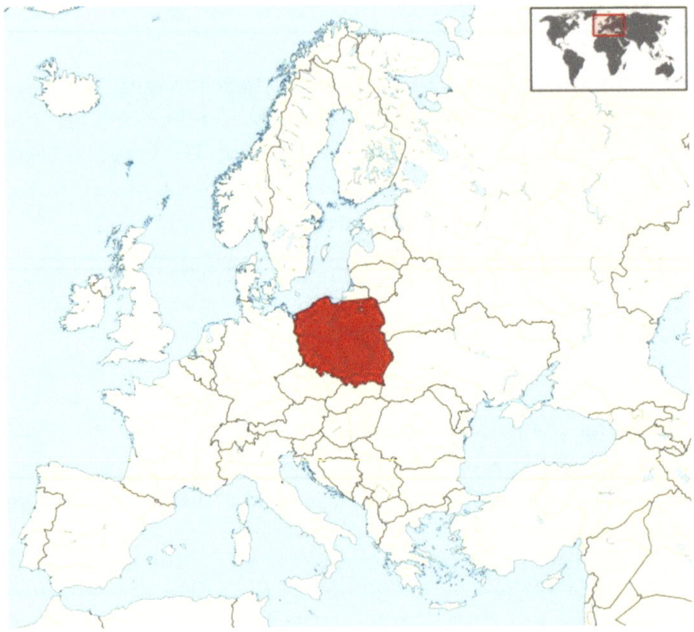

Figure 1. Poland compared to the rest of the world.

Every card was entered in the database created by us in the Excel program and statistically processed. The collected data underwent statistical analysis for measurable and non-measurable traits. Qualitative traits were also analysed by calculating structure ratios. In the statistical analysis of empirical data, the following tests were used to verify hypotheses on the independence of two qualitative traits in the population: Pearson's χ^2 significance test for qualitative variables and χ^2 test with Yates' correction.

Children with an injury accounted for 30.6% of patients from the territory of the Łódzkie region who presented to the Department of Paediatric Emergency Medicine at Maria Konopnicka Memorial University Teaching Hospital No. 4 in Łódź over the year.

Boys decidedly predominated among the injured (60.3%), $p < 0.001$.

Almost 80% of children with an injury were those >5 years of age. No relationship was observed between the child's sex and age, $p > 0.05$.

Prehospital medical aid was the most commonly administered to children by emergency medical service teams (42.7%), less often by a PC physician (28.1%) and other hospitals (23%), and the least commonly by a school nurse (6.1%).

In the study group, children with an injury most often necessitated out-patient treatment (67.1%).

Among children who sustained an injury, traumas to the head (42.1%), upper extremities (32.2%) and lower extremities (19.9%) were noted. Injuries to the abdomen (2.5%), spine (2.1%), chest (1.7%) and neck (1.1%) were less often observed.

In children with a head injury, superficial traumas to the head predominated (53.3%), head wounds (24.3%) and concussions (20.3%) were less common, and fractures of the cranial bones (2.1%) were the least common.

As for children with other bodily injuries, blunt traumas to the neck, superficial chest, abdomen and spine injuries predominated.

Among children in whom upper extremity injuries were observed, traumas to the forearm were the most (42.7%) and to the carporadial joint the least (1.3%) common.

In the group of children with injuries to the lower extremity, ankle joint traumas (26.2%) were the most and traumas within the pelvis, hip joint and kneecap were the least often (1.7%) found.

Burns were the reason for presenting to the Department for 79 out of 1493 patients, which accounted for 5.3% of all children. They were the most often caused by a thermal factor (77 patients), while a chemical burn was found in 1 and an electric burn in 1 child, respectively.

In the group of 1493 children administered first medical aid by different healthcare entities indications for pain management were found in 489 children (32.75%).

Among children who required analgesia, only 159 children (32%) received analgesics, while 223 children (46%) did not receive any and there was no information about analgesia in medical records of 107 patients (22%) (**Figure 2**).

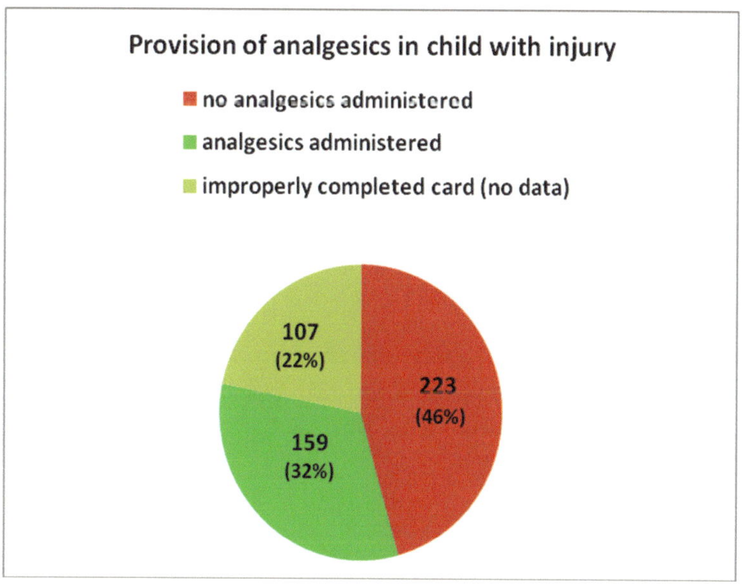

Figure 2. Provision of analgesics in children who sustained injuries.

The provision of analgesics in children with injuries by different healthcare entities is shown in **Table 1**.

Provision of analgesics	**Healthcare entity**							
	Emergency medical service team		**School nurse**		**PC physician**		**Another hospital**	
	Number of children	**Structure ratio [%]**	**Number of children**	**Structure ratio [%]**	**Number of children**	**Structure ratio [%]**	**Number of children**	**Structure ratio [%]**
No analgesics administered	92	44.44	6	40.00	47	49.47	78	45.35
Analgesics administered	104	50.24	8	53.33	15	15.79	32	18.60
No information in the patient transfer card	11	5.31	1	6.67	33	34.74	62	36.05
Total	207	100.00	15	100.00	95	100.00	172	100.00
Statistical analysis	$chi^2_{Pearson}$ test = 87.33 $p < 0.001$; chi^2_{MV} test = 96.30 $p < 0.001$							

Note: statistical analysis did not consider the school nurse.

Table 1. Pain management in the study group.

The performed statistical analysis indicates that all the examined healthcare entities failed to administer analgesics in over 40% of cases (due to their scarce number, patients managed by school nurses were not taken into account). The lack of information about the administration of analgesics in the patient transfer card is also a matter of concern. That was significantly more common in children referred for treatment by a PC physician (34.7%) and patients referred by other hospitals (36%), $p < 0.001$, while that was the least common in children brought to the Department by emergency medical service teams (5.3%)—chi-square$_{Pearson}$ test = 87.33 $p < 0.001$; chi-squared$_{MV}$ test = 96.30 $p < 0.001$ (**Table 1**).

Among children who did not receive analgesics, children with upper extremity fractures—92 cases (41%) and lower extremity fractures—21 cases (9%) predominated. Detailed characteristics of injuries in children who were not provided with analgesics (despite indications) are presented in **Table 2**.

Location of injuries	**Injury, contusion**	**Wound**	**Fracture**	**Dislocation**	**Sprain**	**Burn**
Head	18	14	1	0	0	2
Neck	2	1	0	0	0	0

Location of injuries	Injury, contusion	Wound	Fracture	Dislocation	Sprain	Burn
Chest	3	0	0	0	0	4
Spine	2	0	2	0	0	0
Abdomen	3	0	0	0	0	1
Upper extremity	14	7	**92**	5	0	3
Lower extremity	8	11	**21**	1	4	4

Table 2. Characteristics of injuries in children who were not provided with analgesics n = 223.

In the group of 1493 children administered first medical aid by different healthcare entities transport immobilisation of sustained osteoarticular system injuries was required by 614 children (41.1%). 383 children (62.4%) were properly immobilised for transport, whereas 110 children (17.9%) presented to the Department with no transport immobilisation of fractures, dislocations or sprains. In 121 cases (19.7%), there was no information about applied transport immobilisation in the patient transfer card (**Figure 3**).

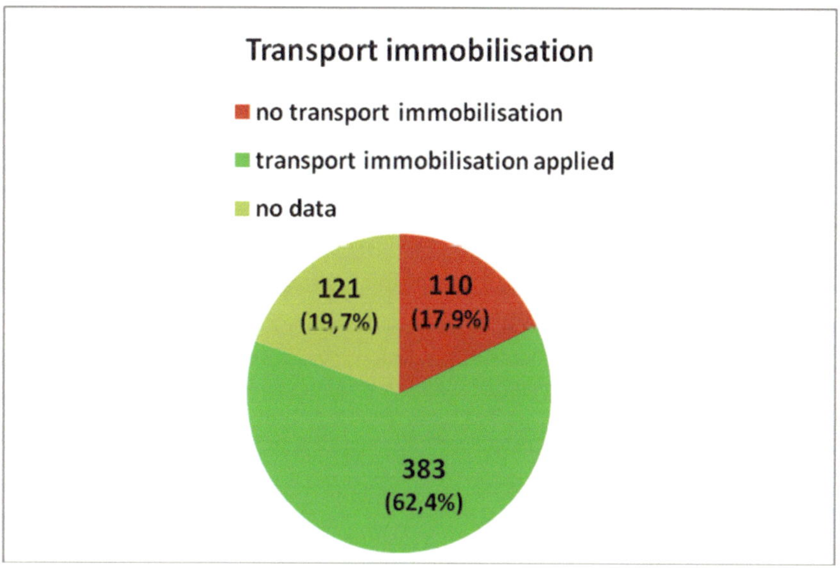

Figure 3. Application of transport immobilisation in children with injury.

Among 383 children immobilised for transport, 261 children (68.1%) were properly and 39 children (10.2%) improperly immobilised. In 83 children (21.7%), it was impossible to determine the quality of applied immobilisation (**Table 3**).

Transport immobilisation	Healthcare entity							
	Emergency medical service team		School nurse		PC physician		Another hospital	
	Number of children	Structure ratio [%]	Number of children	Structure ratio [%]	Number of children	Structure ratio [%]	Number of children	Structure ratio [%]
Application of transport immobilisation	179	72.18	60	84.51	49	39.84	95	55.23
No transport immobilisation	48	19.35	10	14.08	32	26.02	20	11.63
No information in the patient transfer card	21	8.47	1	1.41	42	34.14	57	33.14
Total	248	100.00	71	100.00	123	100.00	172	100.00
Statistical analysis	$chi^2_{Pearson}$ test = 61.92 p<0.001; chi^2_{MV} test = 66.81 p<0.001							
Note: statistical analysis did not consider the school nurse.								

Table 3. Healthcare entity and osteoarticular system immobilisation.

The regularity of transport immobilisation applied in the studied group of children was analysed taking into account the healthcare entity which applied such immobilisation (**Table 4**).

Regularity of transport immobilisation	Healthcare entity							
	Emergency medical service team		School nurse		PC physician		Another hospital	
	Number of children	Structure ratio [%]	Number of children	Structure ratio [%]	Number of children	Structure ratio [%]	Number of children	Structure ratio [%]
Properly applied immobilisation	126	70.39	51	85.00	30	61.22	54	56.84
Improperly applied immobilisation	18	10.06	4	6.66	5	10.21	12	12.63
Appraisal impossible	35	19.55	5	8.34	14	28.57	29	30.53
Total	179	100.00	60	100.00	49	100.00	95	100.00
Statistical analysis	$chi^2_{Pearson}$ test = 41.14 p < 0.001; chi^2_{MV} test = 42.11 p < 0.001							
Note: statistical analysis did not consider the school nurse.								

Table 4. Healthcare entity and regularity of osteoarticular system immobilisation.

The carried out statistical analysis, which due to their scarce number did not take into account patients managed by school nurses, indicated that transport immobilisation in children who required that was most commonly applied by emergency medical service teams, followed by hospital emergency departments/emergency rooms of other hospitals and PC physicians. Those observations were statistically confirmed: $\text{chi-squared}_{\text{Pearson}}$ test = 61.92 $p < 0.001$; $\text{chi-squared}_{\text{MV}}$ test = 66.81 $p < 0.001$.

It should also be noted that transport immobilisation was abandoned by emergency medical service teams in about 20%, by PC physicians in over 26% and by other hospitals in about 11% of cases.

Transport immobilisation was significantly more often properly applied by emergency medical service teams (70.4%) and PC physician (61.2%). On the other hand, only half of the patients from other hospitals presented to the Department properly immobilised (56.9%). Those observations were statistically confirmed: $\text{chi-squared}_{\text{Pearson}}$ test = 41.14 $p < 0.001$; $\text{chi-squared}_{\text{MV}}$ test = 42.11 $p < 0.001$.

It is worth noticing that in the case of one-third children referred to the Department by a PC physician or from other hospitals there was no information about applied transport immobilisation in medical records. It should also be noted that there was no information about the regularity of transport immobilisation in patients transferred by other healthcare entities in almost 30% of cases, while it was known that children had had transport immobilisation applied as such a note had been made in the patient transfer card (Tables **3** and **4**).

Among children who were not immobilised for their transport to the Department, children with upper extremity fractures—33 cases (30%) and lower extremity fractures—14 cases (12.7%) predominated. Children with contusions of various regions of the body—41 cases (37.2%) and sprains within the ankle joint—13 children (11.8%) were also referred to the Department. Detailed characteristics of injuries in children without transport immobilisation are shown in **Table 5**.

Location of injuries	Injury, contusion	Wound	Fracture	Dislocation	Sprain
Head	12	0	3	0	0
Neck	0	0	0	0	0
Chest	2	0	0	0	0
Spine	2	0	2	0	0
Abdomen	3	0	0	0	0
Upper extremity	9	2	**33**	0	0
Lower extremity	13	0	**14**	2	13

Table 5. Characteristics of injuries in children without transport immobilisation n = 110.

Examples of improper transport immobilisation in children who presented to the Department referred by different healthcare entities are shown in Figures **4** and **5**.

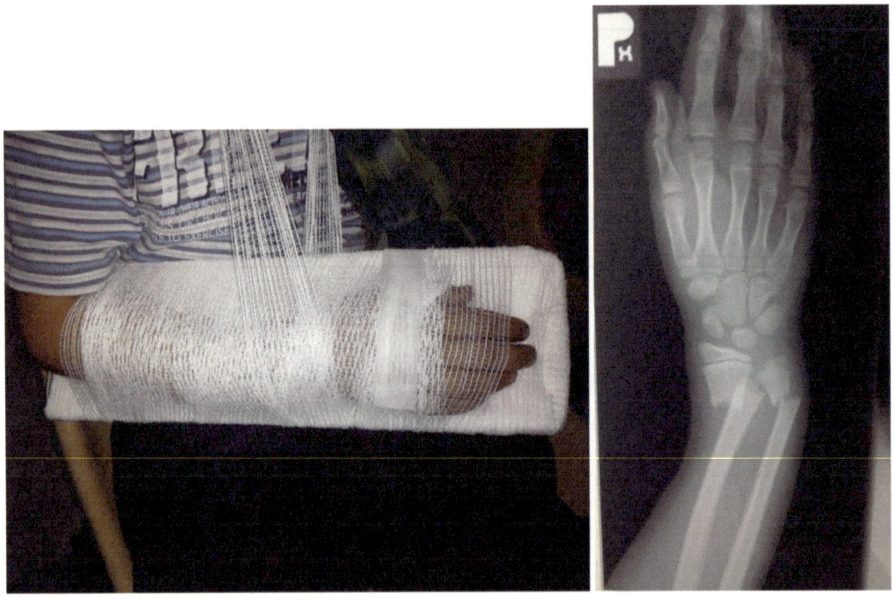

Figure 4. Transport immobilisation in a boy with displaced fractures of both forearm bones.

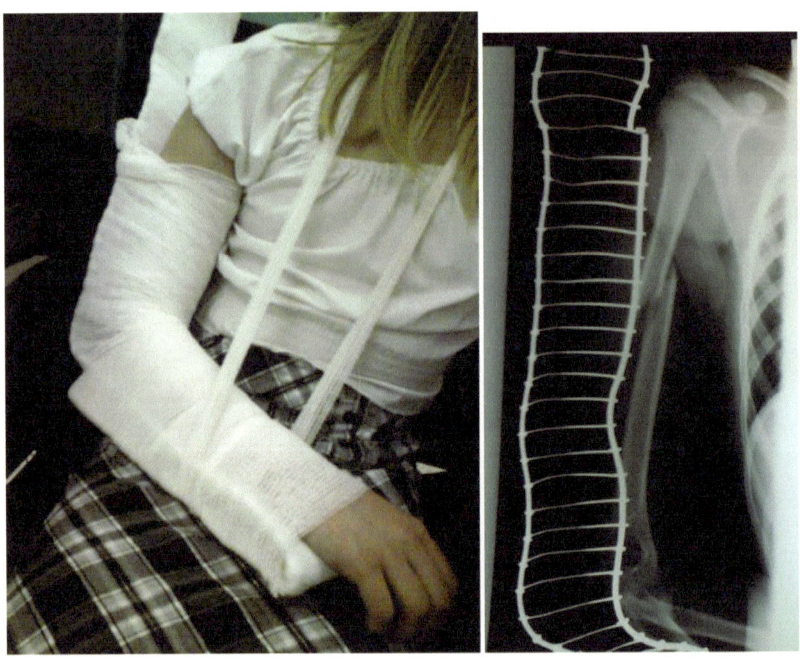

Figure 5. Transport immobilisation in a girl with a humeral bone fracture—bandage fixing the splint to the arm ends at the height of the fracture crevice.

Among 1493 children who were prehospitally managed by different healthcare entities, the integrity of the skin was breached due to an injury in 372 children (24.9%). The medical management of wounds, abrasions or burns in children with an injury is shown in **Figure 6**. Among children not provided with dressing, children with head traumas—15 cases (45%), upper and lower extremity injuries—6 children (18.2%) and burns of different body regions—12 children (36%) predominated.

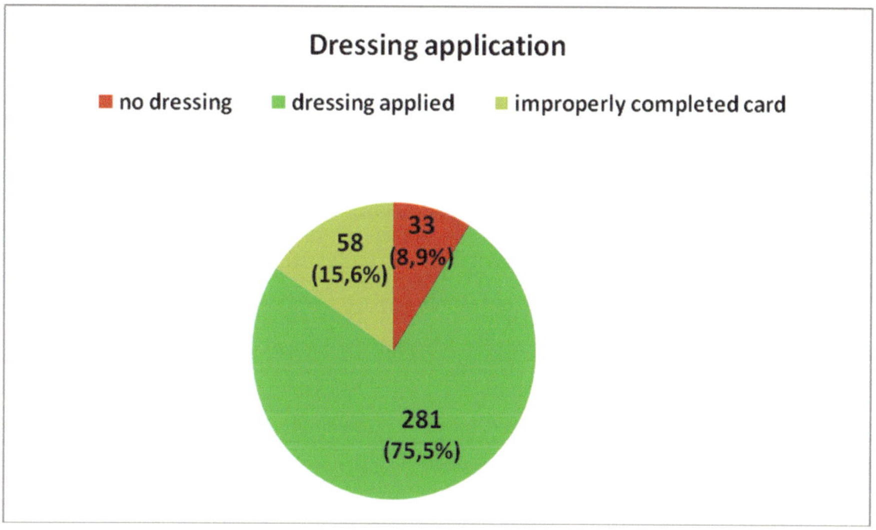

Figure 6. Medical management of wounds, abrasions and burns in the study group.

Among 281 children with dressed integumentary traumas, dressing was properly applied in 260 cases (92.5%), improperly applied dressing was observed in 5 children (1.8%), while no assessment of dressing regularity was noted in 16 cases (5.7%) (**Table 6**).

Wound management	Healthcare entity							
	Emergency medical service team		School nurse		PC physician		Another hospital	
	Number of children	Structure ratio [%]	Number of children	Structure ratio [%]	Number of children	Structure ratio [%]	Number of children	Structure ratio [%]
Dressing applied	174	82.86	10	100.00	42	55.26	55	72.37
No dressing	16	7.62	0	0.00	13	17.11	4	5.26
No information in the patient transfer card	20	9.52	0	0.00	21	27.63	17	22.37
Total	210	100.00	10	100.00	76	100.00	76	100.00

Wound management	Healthcare entity							
	Emergency medical service team		School nurse		PC physician		Another hospital	
	Number of children	Structure ratio [%]	Number of children	Structure ratio [%]	Number of children	Structure ratio [%]	Number of children	Structure ratio [%]
Statistical analysis	$chi^2_{Pearson}$ test = 26.67 $p < 0.001$; chi^2_{MV} test = 25.75 $p < 0.001$							

Note: statistical analysis did not consider the school nurse.

Table 6. Analysis of wound management regularity depending on the healthcare entity.

The regularity of dressing applied in the studied group of children was analysed taking into account the healthcare entity which applied such dressing (**Table 7**).

Regularity of wound management	Healthcare entity							
	Emergency medical service team		School nurse		PC physician		Another hospital	
	Number of children	Structure ratio [%]	Number of children	Structure ratio [%]	Number of children	Structure ratio [%]	Number of children	Structure ratio [%]
Properly applied dressing	166	95.40	10	100.00	37	88.10	47	85.45
Improperly applied dressing	1	0.57	0	0.00	2	4.76	2	3.64
Appraisal impossible	7	4.03	0	0.00	3	7.14	6	10.91
Total	174	100.00	10	100.00	42	100.00	55	100.00
Statistical analysis	$\text{chi-squared}_{Pearson}$ test = 23.15 $p < 0.001$; chi-squared_{MV} test = 24.11 $p < 0.001$							

Note: statistical analysis did not consider the school nurse.

Table 7. Analysis of wound management regularity depending on the healthcare entity.

Although the statistical analysis indicated significantly common proper management of wounds and integumentary injuries, irregularities of that management were observed. Detailed information is shown in Tables **6** and **7**.

In the study group, 124 out of 1493 children (8.3%) necessitated prehospital IV access provision for the intravenous administration of medications or fluids. Among those 124 children, a majority—116 (93.5%) patients—were provided with a peripheral venous catheter, while IV access was not provided in 5 children (4%), and there was no information about IV access in the patient transfer card in 3 children. Among children provided with IV access, irregularities were observed in 2 cases. They consisted in placing a peripheral venous catheter on the fractured extremity in one case and improper securing of IV access in the other (**Figure 7**).

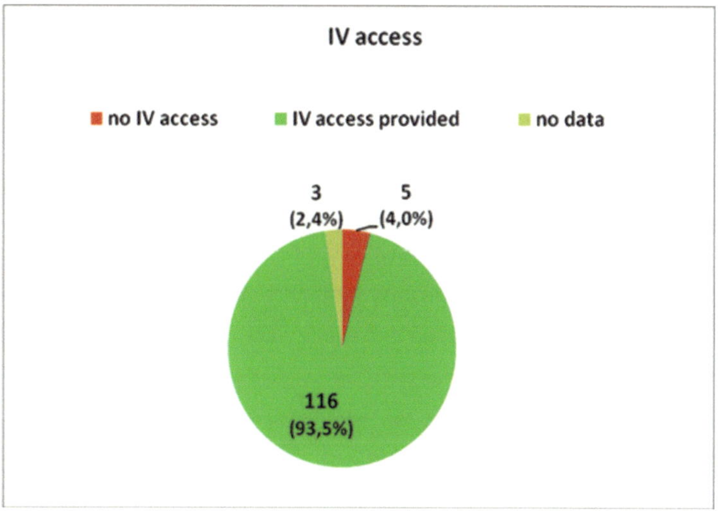

Figure 7. Provision of IV access in the studied population.

Prehospital aid properly administered to the child with an injury significantly affects the prognosis and fate of the patient. Therefore, the knowledge of the rules of management and administration of first aid to the child with bodily injuries is essential to every physician, nurse and paramedic working in the emergency medical service system and primary healthcare.

Own experience and data from the world literature indicate that prehospital medical aid administered to the child with an injury is not always proper. Irregularities most often concern the manner of transport immobilisation and pain management in children with fractures within the osteoarticular system and in children with burns [25, 33, 34]. Main barriers limiting the administration of analgesics (morphine) to children with an injury include difficulty with pain severity assessment in the child, lack of the patient's/legal guardian's consent to receiving analgesics and difficulty with providing IV access [25–27].

Our own study evaluating the manner of administering prehospital aid to the child with an injury by different healthcare entities was based on the observation of 1493 cases.

Boys significantly predominated girls in the study group. The male to female ratio among children was 1.52:1, $p < 0.001$. Similar observations were made by other authors unanimously emphasising that the higher incidence of injuries in boys arises from their increased cognitive activity [5, 13, 35].

The age in the study group ranged from 1 day to 18 years (the median age was 11.4 years, and the mean age was 11.2 years). It was noted that, similarly to other studies in Poland and the world, over 50% of injuries occurred in children aged 5–14 years, $p < 0.001$, which may result from very intense activity and curiosity about the world as well as children's lack of ability to evaluate threatening dangers during play [3, 9, 35].

In the studied group of children prehospital medical aid was most commonly administered by emergency medical service teams (42.7%) and the least commonly by a school nurse (6%), although school was often the place where an injury was sustained. The phenomenon stems from the fact that an emergency medical service team not only administers first medical aid but also ensures professional transport to a hospital emergency department.

When comparing how the administration of prehospital aid to the child with an injury is organised in Poland and the world, some similarities can be observed. In the United States and Canada, when emergency medical service teams are called, prehospital aid is most often administered by emergency medical technicians of the first and second level, paramedics, nurses and the least commonly—physicians [36]. In Poland, in emergency medical service teams, aid is mostly administered by paramedics, and slightly less often—by nurses and physicians.

Among injuries in the children in the study group head injuries were more often observed than in studies by other authors (the study group: 42.1% *vs.* studies of the National Hospital Ambulatory Medical Care Survey ED files: 23.1%), whereas the incidence of extremity injuries was similar to observations by other authors. The predominance of head injuries over extremity injuries observed in our study results from the customary referral of every child with a head injury to the surgeon by the paediatrician. Also, similarly to reports by other authors, minor head injuries predominated among injuries [33, 37, 38].

Neck injuries were rarely found in children and those were mainly blunt traumas and integumentary wounds. Chest and abdominal injuries were slightly more often observed. Among patients who sustained chest injuries, those were mostly superficial chest injuries, with chest wounds and rib fractures being less common. Similarly, in children who suffered an abdominal injury superficial abdominal injuries predominated, while crotch and external genitals or parenchymatous organs injuries were less often observed.

Damage to the upper and lower extremity was among the most common consequences of injuries in children. Our own study indicated that, similarly to the study by Erik M. Hedstrom of Sweden, the most common fracture within the upper extremity was the fracture of the forearm bones, whereas the fracture of the femoral bone shaft was the most common lower extremity injury [3, 15, 38].

The analysis of the management of children with an injury by different healthcare entities showed that a majority of children (72%) were properly administered prehospital medical aid. However, some oversights were found in medical management concerning the administration of analgesics, lack or irregularities of applied transport immobilisation and irregularities in the dressing of integumentary injuries.

Main irregularities observed in 'post-traumatic' children included the lack of the appropriate pain management of children with an injury. As indicated by our own study, pain relief efforts were made in merely 32.5% of children with indications for pain management. Almost a half of patients (45.6%) did not receive any analgesics despite indications. Among children who did not receive analgesics, children with upper extremity fractures (41%) and lower extremity fractures (9.5%) predominated. Similarly to the study by Rawlins [39], we noted the lack of pain management in 6.3% of children with burns. According to the American Academy of Pediatrics and American Pain Society, main barriers to managing pain in children include as follows: the myth that newborns and children feel milder pain than adults, lack of appropriate assessment of the presence of pain, lack of knowledge of pain management and fear of side effects of analgesia (particularly respiratory system depression) [23, 24, 26]. It arises from the study performed by physicians of the paediatric emergency department in Auckland that the fear of causing to the child pain connected with injection resulted in the lack of administration of analgesics [28]. Similar observations were made by the Toronto team [36]. Researchers from the United States also noted that abandoning the administration of analgesics was not associated with the specialty of physician providing aid [26].

Another reservation as to the management of children with an injury regarded the transport immobilisation of children with osteoarticular system injuries. The world and Polish literature offers few studies dedicated to that issue [29, 30]. Out of 614 children requiring transport immobilisation, immobilisation was applied in only 62.4% of cases, out of which in 90% properly. On the other hand, 17.9% of the injured children presented to the Department with no transport immobilisation of fractures, dislocations or sprains, while in 19.7% of cases, there was no information about applied transport immobilisation in the patient transfer card. Among children with improperly applied transport immobilisation, the irregularity of immobilisation concerned the extent of immobilisation and sloppy securing of the transport splint on the injured extremity.

The irregularity of applied transport immobilisation was observed mainly in children with fractures within the osteoarticular system of the upper extremity. Immobilisation irregularities were most common in children with forearm bones' fractures (improper extent), clavicular fractures (sloppy bandaging of the extremity to the chest), humeral fractures (improper extent) and within the hand (2 children—incorrect securing with bandage). Irregularities were also observed in children with lower extremity fractures (improper extent, sloppy securing). There were also cases of improper securing of children after traffic accidents during transport (*e.g.* lack of the cervical collar and incorrect laying on the spinal board (only three straps without side head supports)). The lack of transport immobilisation and its irregularity can be explained by both the lack of knowledge of the proper extent of injured extremity immobilisation and lack of awareness of the fact that properly applied transport immobilisation not only protects against additional injuries but is also a basic method of pain management in the child with an injury within the osteoarticular system. The child with a properly immobilised injured extremity suffers less. Sloppiness in applying transport immobilisation may result from the lack of appreciation of the importance of that medical procedure. During classes, students think that the proper application of transport immobilisation is a very simple task and are not interested enough in that issue. The lack of transport immobilisation may also result from erroneous consideration that handling the child when applying immobilisation may be painful to the child. The lack of medical equipment used to immobilise the extremity which is properly adjusted to the size of the child may also be among reasons behind the lack of the transport immobilisation of the child.

The manner of the dressing of wounds and burns in the study group was also questionable as the lack of dressing was found in 8.9% of patients, improper dressing of a wound—in isolated cases and lack of information about dressing in medical records—in 15.6% of cases. Irregularities in wound dressing concerned burn wounds.

Oversights in administering prehospital aid to children with an injury and gaps in medical records concerned all the studied healthcare entities. Observations concerning neglect while administering first aid to the child with an injury by emergency medical services were described by other authors too [28].

3. Conclusions

1. The management of the child with an injury in the Łódzkie region is unsatisfactory.
2. Despite the training of physicians, nurses and paramedics in the management of paediatric injuries, the lack of analgesic provision is still encountered in almost half of the patients, irregularities in transport immobilisation—in about 10% of the patients and irregularities in wound management and IV access provision—in isolated cases. In one-fourth of the cases, gaps in medical records were also noted.
3. The observed irregularities indicate that it is necessary to intensify training related to medical aid for children after injuries and supplement equipment adjusted to the size of the child available in emergency medical service teams, primary care physicians' surgeries and surgeries at schools.

Author details

Anna Rutkowska* and Grażyna Skotnicka-Klonowicz

*Address all correspondence to: anna.rutkowska@umed.lodz.pl

Central Clinical Hospital, Medical University of Lodz, Poland, Pediatric Center, Maria Konopnicka Memorial

References

[1] Sethi D, Towner E, Vincenten J, Segui- Gomez M, Racioppi F. Europen report on child injury prevention. World Healf Organiyation 2008, chapter 1. 2008;1–22.

[2] Krikwood G, Parekh N, Pollock AM. Preventing injury in children and adolescents. Trauma 2010; 12:221–238.

[3] Tandon T, Shaik M, Modi N. Paediatric trauma epidemiology in an urban scenario in India. Journal of Orthopedic Surgery 2007; 15(1):41–45.

[4] Finkel MD. Public health in the 21st century,Volume 1 global issues in public health, Praeger, California 2011 p.29–46

[5] Ha G, Jeon MJ, Sakong J. Analysis of causes of injuries among children in Daegu, Korea. Korean Journal of Pediatric 2010;53(11):942–950.

[6] Okłot K. Injuries bone joints in children Chapter 1—distinct in structure and principles of treatment of injuries osteoarticular system in children, Publisher PZWL, Warsaw, 1999; 3–61.

[7] Sengoelge M, Hasselberg M, Laflamme L. Child home injury mortality in Europe: a 16—country analysis. European Journal of Public Health Volume 21, Issue 2, April 2010 p.166–170

[8] Amour-Marshall J, Wolfe J, Richardson E, Karanikolos M, McKee M. Childhood deaths from injuries: trends and inequalities in Europe. European Journal of Public Health 2012 22 (1)p. 1–6.

[9] Żyniewicz H, Marcinkowski JT Accidents and injuries in children and adolescents in the light materials ambulance in Poznan. Yearbooks Pomeranian Medical University in Szczecin TOM LI Supplement 1, 2005; 51:147–150.

[10] Nogalski A, Lubek T. The consequences of trauma in children in Lublin province—population studies. Polish Journal of Emergency Medicine 2008; 1:41–49.

[11] Suominem JS, Pakarinen MP, Kääriäinen S, Impinen A, Vartianen E, Helenius I. Hospital treated pediatric injuries are increasing in Finland—a population based study between 1997 and 2006. Scandinavian Journal of Surgery 2011; 100:129–135.

[12] Pearson J, Stone DH. Pattern of injury mortality by age-group in children aged 0–14 years in Scotland, 2002–2006, and its implications for prevention. BMC Paediatrics 2009; 9–26.

[13] UNICEF, World Health Organization. Child and adolescent injury prevention. Global call for Action. 2005:1–14.

[14] Concise Statistical Yearbook Of Poland, central statistical off, Warsaw 2010

[15] Hedström EM, Svensson O, Bergström U, Michno P. Epidemiology of fractures In children and adolescents. Acta Orthopaedica 2010; 81(1):148–153.

[16] MacKenzie EJ. Epidemiology of injuries: current trends and future challenges. Epidemiologic Reviews 2000; 22(1):112–119.

[17] Kleszczyński J, Nabzdyk A. Injuries In Childeren. In: Gula P, Machała W (Eds). Procedure prehospital in body injuries. Medical Publishing PZWL 2015; 323 - 343

[18] Łapoć M, Ciechomski M, Mayzner-Zawadzka E. Pre-hospital care for patients with severe injuries. Intensive and Emergency Medicine 2003; 6(1):29–34.

[19] European Resuscitation Council, Polish Resuscitation Council. Guidelines for Resuscitation 2010 Section 6 Advanced Life Support in Children, Kraków 2010; 181–209.

[20] Daniel M, Borkowska M. The role of emergency medicine in the first aid treatment of burns in children. Yearbook of Pediatric Trauma Surgery 2004; 8(XXXII):99–101.

[21] Strużyna J. First aid in burns at the scene. In: Strużyna J. Burns in disasters and mass events. Medical Publishing PZWL Warsaw 2004; 175–211

[22] King C, Henreting F M. Podręczny atlas emergency procedures in children. And Polish edition, edited by Julius Jakubaszki. Chapter 56. Dressings rail restraints. Medical publisher Uraban & Ground Wrocław 2003; 311–326.

[23] American Academy Of Pediatrics, American Pain Society. The assessment and management of acute pain in infants, children, and adolescents. Pediatrics 2001; 108(3): 793–797.

[24] Mayzner-Zawdzaka E, Błaszyk B, Serednicki W, Dobrogowski J, Wordliczek J, Zawadzki A. In: Proceedings analgesic injuries. Chapter 12 Selected recommendations proceedings anesthesia scientific editor Ewa Mayzner -Zawadzka, Dariusz Kossan, Warsaw PZWL 2008 pp. 97–107.

[25] Zempsky WT, Cravero JP. Relief of pain and anxiety in pediatric patients in emergency medical system. Pediatrics 2004; 114(5):1348–1356.

[26] Brown JC, Klein EJ, Lewis CW, Johnston BD, Cummings P. Emergency department analgesia for fracture pain. Annals of Emergency Medicine 2003; 42(2):197–205.

[27] Hennes H, Kim MK, Pirrallo RG. Prehospital pain management: a comparison of providers perceptions and practices. Prehospital Emergency Care 2005; 9(1):32–39.

[28] Wathins N. Peadiatric prehospital analgesia in Auckland. Emergency Medicine Australas 2006; 18(1):51–56.

[29] Rogovik AL, Goldman RD. Prehospital use of analgesics at home or en route to the hospital in children with extremity injuries. American Journal of Emergency Medicine (2007); 25:400–405.

[30] Spain D. Early management of upper limb fractures in general practice. Australian Family Physician 2004; 33(3):105–109.

[31] Swor R, McEachin CM, Seguin D, Grall KH. Prehospital pain management in children suffering traumatic injury. Prehospital Emergency Care 2005; 1–9.

[32] Nagaraja J, Menkedick J, Phelan KJ, Ashley P, Zhang X, Lanphear BP. Deaths from residential injuries in US children and adolescents, 1985–1997. Pediatrics 2005; 116(2)p. 454–461

[33] Ashworth HL, Cubison TC, Gilbert PM. Treatment before transfer: the patient with burns. Emergency Medicine Journal 2001; 18(5):349–351.

[34] Singer AJ, Thode HC. National analgesia prescribing patterns in emergency department patients with burns. The Journal of Burn Care & Rehabilitation 2002; 23(6):361–365.

[35] Sharma M, Lahoti BK, Khandelwal G, Mathur RK, Sharma SS, Ashok L. Epidemiological trends of pediatric trauma: a single—center study of 791 patients. Journal of Indian Association of Pediatric Surgeons 2011; 16(3):88–92.

[36] Rogovik AL, Goldman RD. Prehospital use of analgesics at home or en route to the hospital in children with extremity injuries. American Journal of Emergency Medicine 2007; 25:400–405.

[37] Singh S, Smith GA, Fields SK, McKenzie LB. Gymnastics-related injuries to children treated in emergency departments in the United States, 1990–2005. Pediatrisc Official Journal of the American Academy of Pediatrics 2008; 121(4):954–960.

[38] Rusck W, Pop T, Jarochowicz S, Cieplińska E, Glista J. The most common injuries upper and lower limbs in children and adolescents. Overview of the Medical University of Rzeszow and the National Drug Institute in Warsaw, Rzeszów 2010; 4:427–434.

[39] Rawlins JM, Khan AA, Shenton AF, Sharpe DT. Epidemiology and outcome analysis of 208 children with burns attending an emergency department. Pediatric Emergency Care 2007; 23(5):289–293.

Chapter 3

Managing Pain with Laser Acupuncture

Szu-Ying Wu, Chun-En Kuo, Yu-Chiang Hung and
Wen-Long Hu

Additional information is available at the end of the chapter

http://dx.doi.org/10.5772/62863

Abstract

According to the theory of traditional Chinese medicine, Qi flows through the body along specific paths known as meridians. Any disturbance in Qi evokes a Ying–Yang imbalance in the body, and consequently leads to disease. Pain results from blood stasis and Qi stagnation. Laser acupuncture (LA), first introduced clinically in the 1970s, combines the advantages of traditional acupuncture and modern laser medicine and has been applied for the treatment of various diseases. Here, we investigated studies on the use of LA for pain management according to current evidence. Articles including English keywords related to the use of LA for pain, published between January 2006 and August 2015 were sourced from PubMed, Medline, and Cochrane Library databases. On the basis of these papers, we explored the modern applications, mechanisms, and analgesic effects of LA. LA integrates the positive effects of acupuncture and low-level laser therapy, and is therefore effective in activating blood and in moving Qi. LA relieves pain through both anti-inflammatory and analgesic effects. No adverse effects or complications resulting from LA were reported in the literature. In the hands of an experienced physician, LA can be a useful and safe method for pain management.

Keywords: laser acupuncture, low-level laser therapy, acupuncture, pain, traditional Chinese medicine

1. Introduction

Although written accounts of acupuncture date back over 2000 years, archaeological evidence suggests more than 3000 years of practice. According to the principles of traditional Chinese medicine (TCM), energy (or Qi) flows through the body along specific paths known as meridians. Balanced Qi contributes to the maintenance of good health. On the other hand, any disturbance in Qi results in an energy imbalance in the body. This imbalance, either an excess or a deficiency, may then result in disease [1]. Both blood stasis and Qi stagnation will lead to pain [2]. In 1996, the World Health Organization (WHO) confirmed 64 indications for acupuncture treatment. Acupuncture treats the underlying diseases by stimulating specific acupuncture points along the meridians. Acupuncture is one of the most common types of alternative treatments for patients who suffer from long-term pain. Moreover, it is a relatively safe procedure with minimal adverse effects [3]. Even though acupuncture has been proven to be effective for many therapeutic applications, metal needling is not widely accepted owing to fear of possible contamination or transcutaneous lesions [4]. Consequently, following the theory of TCM, the use of low-level laser on acupuncture points has been developed as a new therapeutic approach called laser acupuncture (LA) [5, 6].

LA was first introduced clinically in the 1970s [7]. It has been widely studied over several years to turn it into an evidence-based clinical practice. The use of low-intensity and nonthermal laser irradiation stimulation of acupuncture points is an effective alternative to traditional metal needling; it is a safe technique because it is noninvasive and is acceptable to needle-phobic persons. Thus, LA can be used at acupuncture points that require complicated applications of needles [1, 8]. The laser beam is an electromagnetic wave and can stimulate acupuncture points in the human body by depositing energy without causing heating. In contrast to needling, acupuncture points irradiated by a laser beam need to receive sufficient energy to induce a physiological effect at the cellular level based on the principle of "photobiomodulation." The beam excites the relevant channels and activities, regulates the function of organs, and promotes metabolism. Recently, several papers have reported that the decisive factor in the efficacy of LA is the applied dosage [5, 9–11].

Although the mechanisms underlying LA are not well understood, LA is widely applied clinically. LA is also referred to as low-level laser therapy (LLLT), with 0.1–0.5 J/cm^2 deposited per acupuncture point, or 1–4 J/cm^2 per Ashi point [12]. LLLT has an anti-inflammatory function because it can reduce the levels of certain biochemical factors (prostaglandin E2, messenger ribonucleic acid cyclooxygenase-2, interleukin (IL)-1β, and tumor necrosis factor (TNF)-α), neutrophil influx, oxidative stress, edema, and hemorrhaging [13]. Analgesia induced by laser phototherapy is mediated by peripheral opioid receptors [14]. Nevertheless, LA has both local and distant analgesic effects, which may be mediated by different mechanisms. LA combines the advantages of traditional metal-needle acupuncture and LLLT. This chapter on managing pain by LA focuses on how LA may be an alternative method of relieving pain and improving functional outcomes.

2. Review of the clinical literature

Clinical literature in electronic databases—PubMed, Medline, and Cochrane library—was surveyed using the terms "laser acupuncture", "low level laser therapy", and "pain", published from January 2006 to August 2015. All papers had to meet the following criteria: randomized controlled trials (RCTs) that considered a control group (either placebo, sham LA, nonstandard traditional acupuncture, or other therapeutic equipment) and retrospective/prospective clinical studies in which LA/LLLT was used. Studies cited in review articles were also included. Papers published in languages other than English were excluded. Conference abstracts, single-case studies, and paper for which full text was not available were also excluded.

Among the reviewed literature, most studies targeted myofascial pain, fibromyalgia, tendinopathy, radiculopathy, osteoarthritis (OA), low back pain, temporomandibular joint dysfunction (TMD), and headache. These are discussed below.

2.1. Myofascial pain

Kiralp et al. [15] reported a RCT in which 43 patients with myofascial pain were enrolled, and showed the positive effect of LA as compared to prilocaine injection. Eight other RCTs also showed the pain-relieving effect of LA; some of these focused on myofascial pain over the cervical region [16, 17], masseter [18], masticatory muscles [19, 20], trapezius [21, 22], or trigger points [23]. The consistency of these trials highlighted the efficacy of LA in the treatment of myofascial pain.

2.2. Fibromyalgia

Two RCTs showed different results for LA treatment of fibromyalgia [24, 25]. Both of these studies obtained subjective pain presentation using a visual analog scale (VAS), the Fibromyalgia Impact Questionnaire (FIQ), and other measures. Armagan et al. [24] reported positive results of LA for treating the pain of fibromyalgia. The difference between these studies was the dose and power density. Armagan et al. set the parameters of LA to 830 nm, 2 J/point, and 50 mW. These results suggested that the treatment effect of LA was inconclusive in fibromyalgia or that the power density used should be sufficiently high to manage the pain in this disease group.

2.3. Tendinopathy

Two RCTs showed positive results of LA in pain management of lateral epicondylitis (LE) [26, 27], also known as tennis elbow. Emanet et al. [27] reported that even though LA had no short-term advantage over the placebo in patients with LE, there was a significant long-term improvement, especially in functional parameters. Another RCT reported that LA had a treatment effect equal to that of ultrasound [28]. Moreover, a systemic review revealed that applying LLLT to myofascial trigger points of LE patients was an effective treatment for pain reduction and also led to increase in grip force, range of motion (ROM), and weight test [9]. As for tendomyopathy of the masticatory musculature, the pilot study showed inconclusive results because there were few participants [19].

2.4. Radiculopathy

Konstantinovic et al. [29] performed an RCT that enrolled 60 patients with acute neck pain with cervical radiculopathy. After a 3-week LA treatment, VAS, neck movement, neck disability index, and quality of life indicated the positive effect of LA. Radiculopathy of other spinal segments was not reported.

2.5. Osteoarthritis

Among the four RCTs on the use of LA in treating the pain of knee OA, two showed a positive result [30, 31], one was inconclusive [32], and the other one reported efficacy after 2 weeks of treatment but not at the 4-week assessment [33]. However, the RCT showed the inconclusive result for only one point, ST35. An inappropriate dose or insufficient irradiation at a point may be the reason for the poor treatment effect.

2.6. Low back pain

Glazov et al. [34] had reported negative result for the use of LA to relieve low back pain in their study, in which LA was applied to local points of three meridians (Bladder, Gallbladder, and Governor vessel) and Ashi points. Subsequently, Glazov [35] reported another RCT, in which 100 patients with low back pain were enrolled, and found a positive result for pain management with LA. However, the parameter settings used for the second RCT were not described. Therefore, we were not able to determine the differences that contributed to the successful treatment. Nevertheless, further two RCTs showed a positive response for low back pain treated with LA [36, 37].

2.7 Temporomandibular joint disorder

In our literature search, all four RCTs suggested a positive treatment effect for LA in treating the pain associated with TMD [4, 38–40]. Occlusal splinting is the nonsurgical standard treatment for this condition in dental clinics. In two RCTs, LA was found to be as effective as occlusal splinting in relieving TMD-associated pain [39, 40]. LA could be an alternative treatment choice to occlusal splinting. Sattayut and Bradley [41] compared low- and high-grade LA and found that high-grade LA, i.e., 820 nm, 107 J/cm^2, and 300 mW, showed a superior treatment effect. More recently, Hu et al. [42] clearly showed the therapeutic effects of LA in managing treatment-resistant TMD. In our literature review, another two clinical trials revealed the benefit of LA therapy for TMD patients [43, 44].

2.8. Headache

Gottschling et al. [45] reported an RCT in which LA was used to treat headache in children and showed a decrease in the VAS score and monthly hours with headache. Interestingly, the treatment in this study consisted of only four treatment episodes, at a frequency of once a week, yet the improvement of symptoms was excellent. This study also focused on the meridian-based selection of irradiation points. The basic points for patients with frontal headache were LI4 and ST36; for lateral pain, they were TE6 and GB34; for occipital pain, they were SI3 and BL60, and for holocephalic pain, it was GV20. Additional body acupuncture points and ear acupuncture points were chosen individually. The combination of TCM meridian theory with

http://dx.doi.org/10.5772/62863

LA energy treatment seemed to provide a better effect than simply irradiating the tender points.

2.9. Others

Chow et al. [17] reported that chronic neck pain of any etiology could be treated successfully with a program of 14 LA treatments over a period of 7 weeks. Ip and Fu [46] reported a prospective cohort study that proved the treatment efficacy of LA in painful adhesive capsulitis of the shoulder.

3. Conclusions

We have presented evidence supporting the use of LA in the management for various types of pain (Table 1). LA is a noninvasive technique involving the stimulation of traditional acupuncture points with low-intensity laser irradiation. LA has the advantages of being painless and safe as no heat is generated during the procedure, and it is more effective in some medical conditions and requires less time than needle-based acupuncture [47]. No adverse effects or complications resulting from LA have been reported in any study to date. The effectiveness of LA in managing pain depends on the selection of appropriate points and frequencies. Insufficient energy and very few therapeutic sessions will result in ineffective therapy. In conclusion, LA combines the positive effects of traditional Chinese acupuncture and LLLT, and is therefore effective in both activating blood and moving Qi. LA relieves pain through both anti-inflammatory and analgesic effects. As experienced physicians, we should optimize laser parameters, treatment intervals, and long-term follow-up for LA therapy.

Study	Study design	Subjects	Diagnosis	Control	Intervention time	Wavelength	Dose	Power	Irradiation time (s)	Acupoints	Outcome measure	Results
Kıralp et al. [15]	RCT	43	Myofascial pain syndrome	Prilocaine injection	4 weeks (12 sessions)	–	–	–	180	Trigger points in the neck, shoulder, and back muscles	VAS, VPS, pressure pain threshold by pressure algometer	Positive in pressure algometer
Chow et al. [17]	RCT	90	Chronic neck pain	Placebo	7 weeks (14 sessions)	830 nm	0.67 W/cm²	300 mW	30	Tender points	VAS	Positive
Armagan et al. [24]	RCT	32	Fibromyalgia	Placebo	2 weeks (10 sessions)	830 nm	2 J/point	50 mW	60	Tender points	NTP, FIQ, morning stiffness, VSGI, and total myalgia score	Positive
Yurtkuran et al. [30]	RCT	52	Knee OA	Placebo	2 weeks (10 sessions)	904 nm	0.48 J	10 mW	120	SP9	VAS, 50-foot walking time, KC, MTS, WOMAC, NHP	Improvement in KC
Mazzetto et al. [38]	RCT	48	TMD	Placebo	4 weeks (8 sessions)	708 nm	89.7 J/cm²	70 mW	10	One point inside the external auditive duct	VAS	Positive
Matsutani et al. [25]	RCT	20	Fibromyalgia	Stretching plus LLLT versus no laser	End of intervention	830 nm	3 J/cm²	30 mW	–	–	VAS, dolorimetry at tender points, FIQ, SF-36	Negative
Lam and Cheing [26]	RCT	39	Lateral epicondylitis	Placebo	3 weeks (9 sessions)	904 nm	2.4 J/cm²	25 mW	11	Tender points	VAS, DASH questionnaire	Positive
Dundar et al. [16]	RCT	64	Cervical Myofascial pain	Placebo	3 weeks (15 sessions)	830 nm	7 J/point	58 mW	120	Trigger points	VAS, ROM,	Positive

Study	Study design	Subjects	Diagnosis	Control	Intervention time	Wavelength	Dose	Power	Irradiation time (s)	Acupoints	Outcome measure	Results
											neck disability index	
Shen et al. [31]	RCT	48	Knee OA	Combined laser versus red light	3 times/week for 2 weeks then 2 times/week for 4 weeks	650 nm semiconductor laser plus 10.6 μm CO_2 laser	–	–	–	ST35	WOMAC	Positive but in-conclusive difference
Gottschling et al. [45]	RCT	43	Headache in children	Placebo	4 weeks (4 sessions)	830 nm	0.9 J/point	30 mW	30	LI4, ST36; TE6, GB34; SI3, BL60; GV20	VAS; monthly hours with headache	Positive
Shirani et al. [20]	RCT	16	Myofascial pain of masticatory system	Placebo	3 weeks (6 sessions)	660 nm; 890 nm	6.2 J/cm^2; 1 J/cm^2	17.3mW; 9.8 W	180; 600	Tender points	VAS	Positive
Shen et al. [32]	RCT	40	Knee OA	Placebo	4 weeks (12 sessions)	650 nm semiconductor laser plus 10.6 μm CO_2 laser	–	36 mW; 200 mW	1200	ST35	WOMAC	In-conclusive
Glazov et al. [34]	RCT	100	Chronic non-specific low back pain	Placebo	5–10 sessions	830 nm	0.2 J/point	10 mW	20	Points on BL, GB, GV meridians; Ashi points	VAS; ODI; DASS-21; PWI-A	Negative
Carrasco et al. [23]	RCT	60	Myofascial pain	Placebo	4 weeks (8 sessions)	780 nm	25, 60 and 105 J/cm^2	–	–	Trigger point	–	Positive
Zhao et al. [33]	RCT	40	Knee OA	Non-acupoint sham control	4 weeks (12 sessions)	650 nm semiconductor laser plus 10.6 μm CO_2 laser	650 nm laser energy of 43.2 J ; 10.6 μm laser energy of 120 J	36 mW; 200 mW	1200	ST35	WOMAC	Positive after 2 weeks treatment, but not at 4 weeks
Öz et al. [39]	RCT	40	Myofascial pain due to TMD	occlusal splint	5 weeks (10 sessions)	820 nm	3 J/cm^2	300 mW	–	–	VAS	As effective
Katsoulis et al. [19]	Pilot study	11	Tendomyopathy of masticatory musculature	Placebo	3 weeks (6 sessions)	690 nm	40-60 J	40 mW	900	ST6, SI18, SI3, LI4	VAS	In-conclusive
Glazov [35]	RCT	100	Low back pain	Placebo	5–10 sessions	–	–	–	–	–	VAS	Positive
Hotta et al. [43]	Clinical trial	10	TMD	No treatment	10 weeks (10 sessions)	780 nm	35 J/cm^2	70 mW	20	LI4, HT3, ST6, ST7	EMG, VAS	Positive
Konstantinovic et al. [29]	RCT	60	Acute neck pain with cervical radiculopathy	Placebo	3 weeks (15 sessions)	905 nm	2 J/cm^2	12 mW/cm^2	120	Lateral to spinous process and the two next spinal segment	VAS, neck movement, neck disability index, quality of life	Positive
Lee and Han [21]	RCT	24	Myofascial trigger point pain	Placebo	End of intervention	830 nm	386, 771, 1929 J/cm^2	450 mW	1, 2, 5 min	Trigger points	PPT	Positive in 5 min
Emanet et al. [27]	RCT	50	Lateral epicondylitis	Placebo	3 weeks (15 sessions)	905 nm	1 J/cm^2	–	120	Two most sensitive points around the lateral epicondyle	VAS, tenderness, DASH questionnaire, PRTEE test, pain-free grip strength, NHP questionnaire	Positive in long-term evaluation (12 weeks)
Skorupska et al. [28]	RCT	80	Tennis elbow	Ultrasound	10 days with a weekend break (10 sessions)	820 ± 10 nm	1; 5 J/cm^2	400 mW	–	Trigger points	Algometer, VAS, DASH questionnaire, and hand grip strength	Equally effective
Kannan [22]	RCT	45	Myofascial pain of upper trapezius	ultrasound ; ischemic compression	5 days (5 sessions)	904 nm	74 mJ/cm^2	–	30	Trigger points	VAS, provocative pain test, active lateral bending of the cervical spine	Positive
Sattayut and Bradley [41]	RCT	30	Temporomandibular joint disorder	Low-energy-density laser versus high-energy versus placebo	1 week (3 sessions)	820 nm	21.4, 107 J/cm^2	60 mW; 300 mW	–	3 points around TMJ; 3 most tender trigger points	PPT, MOSP, SSI, EMG	Positive in higher energy group
Lin et al. [36]	RCT	60	Low back pain	Placebo	5 days (5 sessions)	808 nm	15 J/cm^2	40 mW	600	BL40; Ashi acupoints	VAS, Ryodoraku	Positive
Ferreira et al. [4]	RCT	40	TMD	Placebo	3 months (12 sessions)	780 nm	112.5 J/cm^2	50 mW	90	ST6, SI19, GB20, GB43, LI4, LR3, NT3, EX-HN3	VAS	Positive
Uemoto et al. [18]	RCT	21	Myofascial pain syndrome of masseter muscle	Anesthetic injection,	8 days (4 sessions)	795 nm	Right: 4 J/cm^2; Left: 8 J/cm^2	80 mW	–	Trigger points	Surface EMG, mouth opening, VAS	Positive

http://dx.doi.org/10.5772/62863

Study	Study design	Subjects	Diagnosis	Control	Intervention time	Wavelength	Dose	Power	Irradiation time (s)	Acupoints	Outcome measure	Results
				dry needling, placebo								
Huang et al. [44]	Clinical trial	20	TMD	Placebo	Once a week till symptom relief or 3 weeks of no improvement	800 nm	100.5 J/cm^2	0.75 W/cm^2	134	ST6, ST7, LI4 and one local Ashi point	VAS	Positive
Demirkol et al. [40]	RCT	30	Myofascial pain due to TMD	occlusal splint; placebo	10 days (10 sessions)	1064 nm	8 J/cm^2	250 mW	20	Trigger points	VAS	As effective as occlusal splint
Hu et al. [42]	Clinical trial	29	Treatment-resistant TMD	–	4 weeks (12 sessions)	810 nm	7.5–26.25 J/cm^2	5 W/cm^2	5 sec (acupoint); 40 sec (Ashi point)	ST7, ST6, LI4 and Ashi point	VAS, MMO	Positive
Shin et al. [37]	RCT	56	Low back pain	Sham laser	1 week (3 sessions)	660 nm	–	50 mW	180	GV3, GV4, GV5, BL23, BL24, BL25, BL40, GB30	VAS, PPT, PGIC, EQ-5D	Positive
Ip and Fu [46]	Prospective cohort study	50	Painful adhesive capsulitis of shoulder	–	8 week (24 sessions)	810 nm	5.4 J/point	20 mW/cm^2	20–30	6 anatomic points; SI11, SI12	Constant Murley shoulder score	Positive

DASH: disabilities of the arm, shoulder, and hand; DASS-21: Depression Anxiety Stress Scale; EMG: electromyography; EQ-5D: Euro-Quality-of-Life Five Dimensions questionnaire; KC: knee circumference; MOSP: maximum mouth opening (MMO) without pain; MTS: medial tenderness score; NHP: Nottingham Health Profile; NTP: number of tender points; ODI: Oswestry Disability Index; PGIC: Patient Global Impression of Change; PPT: pressure pain threshold; PRTEE: Patient-Related Lateral Epicondylitis Evaluation; PWI-A: Personal Wellbeing Index; SF-36: 36-item Short-Form Health Survey; VPS: verbal pain scale; VSGI: global improvement on a verbal scale; WOMAC: Western Ontario and McMaster Universities osteoarthritis index.

Table 1. Summary of clinical studies into pain management with laser acupuncture.

Abbreviations

DASH disabilities of the arm, shoulder and hand

DASS-21 Depression Anxiety Stress Scale

EMG electromyography

EQ-5D Euro-Quality-of-Life Five Dimensions questionnaire

FIQ Fibromyalgia Impact Questionnaire

FIQ Fibromyalgia Impact Questionnaire

KC knee circumference

LA laser acupuncture

LE lateral epicondylitis

LLLT low-level laser therapy

MOSP maximum mouth opening (MMO) without pain

MTS medial tenderness score

NHP Nottingham Health Profile

NTP number of tender points

OA osteoarthritis

ODI Oswestry Disability Index

PGIC Patient Global Impression of Change

PPT pressure pain threshold

PRTEE Patient-Related Lateral Epicondylitis Evaluation

PWI-A Personal Wellbeing Index

RCT randomized controlled trial

ROM active range of motion

SF-36 36-item Short-Form Health Survey

SSI symptom severity index

TCM traditional Chinese medicine

TMD temporomandibular joint (TMJ) disorder

VAS visual analogue scale

VPS verbal pain scale

VSGI global improvement on a verbal scale

WHO World Health Organization

WOMAC Western Ontario and McMaster Universities osteoarthritis index

Author details

Szu-Ying Wu[1], Chun-En Kuo[1], Yu-Chiang Hung[1,2] and Wen-Long Hu[1,3,4*]

*Address all correspondence to: oolonghu@gmail.com

1 Department of Chinese Medicine, Kaohsiung Chang Gung Memorial Hospital and School of Traditional Chinese Medicine, Chang Gung University College of Medicine, Kaohsiung, Taiwan

2 School of Chinese Medicine for Post Baccalaureate, I-Shou University, Kaohsiung, Taiwan

3 Fooyin University College of Nursing, Kaohsiung, Taiwan

4 Kaohsiung Medical University College of Medicine, Kaohsiung, Taiwan

References

[1] Whittaker P. Laser acupuncture: past, present, and future. Lasers in Medical Science. 2004;19(2):69–80.

[2] Bing Z, Hongcai W. Diagnostics of traditional Chinese medicine. 1st ed. London and Philadelphia: Singing Dragon; 2010. 224 p.

[3] Rickards LD. Therapeutic needling in osteopathic practice: An evidence-informed perspective. International Journal of Osteopathic Medicine. 2009;12(1):2–13.

[4] Ferreira LA, de Oliveira RG, Guimarães JP, Carvalho ACP, De Paula MVQ. Laser acupuncture in patients with temporomandibular dysfunction: A randomized controlled trial. Lasers in Medical Science. 2013;28(6):1549–1558.

[5] Baxter GD, Bleakley C, McDonough S. Clinical effectiveness of laser acupuncture: A systematic review. Journal of Acupuncture and Meridian Studies. 2008;1(2):65–82.

[6] Round R, Litscher G, Bahr F. Auricular acupuncture with laser. Evidence-Based Complementary and Alternative Medicine. 2013;2013:984763. doi: 10.1155/2013/984763. 22 pages.

[7] Hill S. Letter: Acupuncture research in the USSR. The American Journal of Chinese Medicine. 1976;4(2):204.

[8] Litscher G. High-tech laser acupuncture is Chinese medicine. Medical Acupuncture. 2008;20(4):245–254.

[9] Chang W-D, Wu J-H, Yang W-J, Jiang J-A. Therapeutic effects of low-level laser on lateral epicondylitis from differential interventions of Chinese-Western medicine: Systematic review. Photomedicine and Laser Surgery. 2010;28(3):327–336.

[10] Peplow PV, Chung T-Y, Baxter GD. Laser photobiomodulation of proliferation of cells in culture: A review of human and animal studies. Photomedicine and Laser Surgery. 2010;28(S1):S3–S40.

[11] Litscher G, Opitz G. Technical parameters for laser acupuncture to elicit peripheral and central effects: State-of-the-art and short guidelines based on results from the Medical University of Graz, the German Academy of Acupuncture, and the scientific literature. Evidence-Based Complementary and Alternative Medicine. 2012;2012:697096. doi: 10.1155/2012/697096. 5 pages.

[12] Wen-Long Hu, Yu-Chiang Hung, I-Ling Hung. Explore Laser Acupuncture's Role. In: Lucy L. Chen, Tsung O. Cheng, editors. Acupuncture in Modern Medicine. 1st ed. Rijeka: InTech; 2013. p. 205-220. ch9.

[13] Bjordal JM, Johnson MI, Iversen V, Aimbire F, Lopes-Martins RAB. Low-level laser therapy in acute pain: A systematic review of possible mechanisms of action and clinical

effects in randomized placebo-controlled trials. Photomedicine and Laser Therapy. 2006;24(2):158–168.

[14] Serra AP, Ashmawi HA. Influence of naloxone and methysergide on the analgesic effects of low-level laser in an experimental pain model. Brazilian Journal of Anesthesiology. 2010;60(3):302–310.

[15] Kiralp MZ, Ari H, Karabekir I, Dursun H. Comparison of low intensity laser therapy and trigger point injection in the management of myofascial pain syndrome. The Pain Clinic. 2006;18(1):63–66.

[16] Dundar U, Evcik D, Samli F, Pusak H, Kavuncu V. The effect of gallium arsenide aluminum laser therapy in the management of cervical myofascial pain syndrome: A double blind, placebo-controlled study. Clinical Rheumatology. 2007;26(6):930–934.

[17] Chow RT, Heller GZ, Barnsley L. The effect of 300mW, 830nm laser on chronic neck pain: A double-blind, randomized, placebo-controlled study. Pain. 2006;124(1):201–210.

[18] Uemoto L, Antonio C Garcia M, Vinicius D Gouvêa C, Vilella OV, Alfaya TA. Laser therapy and needling in myofascial trigger point deactivation. Journal of Oral Science. 2013;55(2):175–181.

[19] Katsoulis J, Ausfeld-Hafter B, Katsoulis K, Blagojevic N, Mericske-Stern R. Laser acupuncture for myofascial pain of the masticatory muscles. A controlled pilot study. Schweiz Monatsschr Zahnmed. 2010;120(3):213-225.

[20] Shirani AM, Gutknecht N, Taghizadeh M, Mir M. Low-level laser therapy and myofacial pain dysfunction syndrome: A randomized controlled clinical trial. Lasers in Medical Science. 2009;24(5):715–720.

[21] Lee JH, Han JT. The dose-dependent effect of an 830-nm, 450-mW low-level laser therapy on the myofacial trigger point of the upper trapezius muscle: A randomized, double-blinded, clinical trial. Journal of Physical Therapy Science. 2011;23(6):933–935.

[22] Kannan P. Management of myofascial pain of upper trapezius: A three group comparison study. Global Journal of Health Science. 2012;4(5): 46-52.

[23] Carrasco TG, Guerisoli LDC, Guerisoli DMZ, Mazzetto MO. Evaluation of low intensity laser therapy in myofascial pain syndrome. CRANIO®. 2009;27(4):243–7.

[24] Armagan O, Tascioglu F, Ekim A, Oner C. Long-term efficacy of low level laser therapy in women with fibromyalgia: A placebo-controlled study. Journal of Back and Musculoskeletal Rehabilitation. 2006;19(4):135–140.

[25] Matsutani L, Marques A, Ferreira E, Assumpção A, Lage L, Casarotto R, et al. Effectiveness of muscle stretching exercises with and without laser therapy at tender points for patients with fibromyalgia. Clinical and Experimental Rheumatology. 2007;25(3): 410–415.

[26] Lam LKY, Cheing GLY. Effects of 904-nm low-level laser therapy in the management of lateral epicondylitis: A randomized controlled trial. Photomedicine and Laser Surgery. 2007;25(2):65–71.

[27] Emanet SK, Altan Lİ, Yurtkuran M. Investigation of the effect of GaAs laser therapy on lateral epicondylitis. Photomedicine and Laser Surgery. 2010;28(3):397–403.

[28] Skorupska E, Lisinski P, Samborski W. The effectiveness of the conservative versus myofascial pain physiotherapy in tennis elbow patients: Double-blind randomized trial of 80 patients. Journal of Musculoskeletal Pain. 2011;20(1):41–50.

[29] Konstantinovic LM, Cutovic MR, Milovanovic AN, Jovic SJ, Dragin AS, Letic MD, et al. Low-level laser therapy for acute neck pain with radiculopathy: a double-blind placebo-controlled randomized study. Pain Medicine. 2010;11(8):1169–1178.

[30] Yurtkuran M, Alp A, Konur S, Özçakir S, Bingol U. Laser acupuncture in knee osteo-arthritis: A double-blind, randomized controlled study. Photomedicine and Laser Therapy. 2007;25(1):14–20.

[31] Shen X-Y, Ding G-H, Wu F, Wang L-Z, Zhao L, Wang M, et al. Effects of 650 nm-10.6 μm combined laser acupuncture-moxibustion on knee osteoarthritis: A randomized, double-blinded and placebo-controlled clinical trial. Journal of Acupuncture and Tuina Science. 2008;6:315–317.

[32] Shen X, Zhao L, Ding G, Tan M, Gao J, Wang L, et al. Effect of combined laser acu-puncture on knee osteoarthritis: A pilot study. Lasers in Medical Science. 2009;24(2): 129–136.

[33] Zhao L, Shen X, Cheng K, Deng H, Ding G, Tan M, et al. Validating a nonacupoint sham control for laser treatment of knee osteoarthritis. Photomedicine and Laser Surgery. 2010;28(3):351–356.

[34] Glazov G, Schattner P, Lopez D, Shandley K. Laser acupuncture for chronic non-specific low back pain: A controlled clinical trial. Acupuncture in Medicine. 2009;27(3): 94–100.

[35] Glazov G. The influence of baseline characteristics on response to a laser acupuncture intervention: An exploratory analysis. Acupuncture in Medicine. 2010;28(1):6–11.

[36] Lin M-L, Wu H-C, Hsieh Y-H, Su C-T, Shih Y-S, Lin C-W, et al. Evaluation of the effect of laser acupuncture and cupping with ryodoraku and visual analog scale on low back pain. Evidence-Based Complementary and Alternative Medicine. 2012;2012:521612. doi: 10.1155/2012/521612. 7 pages.

[37] Shin J-Y, Ku B, Kim JU, Lee YJ, Kang JH, Heo H, et al. Short-Term effect of laser acupuncture on lower back pain: A Randomized, Placebo-Controlled, Double-Blind Trial. Evidence-Based Complementary and Alternative Medicine. 2015;2015:808425. doi: 10.1155/2015/808425. 8 pages.

[38] Mazzetto MO, Carrasco TG, Bidinelo EF, de Andrade Pizzo RC, Mazzetto RG. Low intensity laser application in temporomandibular disorders: A phase I double-blind study. CRANIO®. 2007;25(3):186–92.

[39] Öz S, Gökçen-Röhlig B, Saruhanoglu A, Tuncer EB. Management of myofascial pain: Low-level laser therapy versus occlusal splints. Journal of Craniofacial Surgery. 2010;21(6):1722–1728.

[40] Demirkol N, Sari F, Bulbul M, Demirkol M, Simsek I, Usumez A. Effectiveness of occlusal splints and low-level laser therapy on myofascial pain. Lasers in Medical Science. 2014;30(3):1007–1012.

[41] Sattayut S, Bradley P. A study of the influence of low intensity laser therapy on painful temporomandibular disorder patients. Laser Therapy. 2012;21(3):183–192.

[42] Hu W-L, Chang C-H, Hung Y-C, Tseng Y-J, Hung I-L, Hsu S-F. Laser acupuncture therapy in patients with treatment-resistant temporomandibular disorders. PLoS One. 2014;9(10):e110528.

[43] Hotta PT, Hotta TH, Bataglion C, Bataglion SA, de Souza Coronatto EA, Siéssere S, et al. Emg analysis after laser acupuncture in patients with temporomandibular dysfunction (TMD). Implications for practice. Complementary Therapies in Clinical Practice. 2010;16(3):158–160.

[44] Huang Y-F, Lin J-C, Yang H-W, Lee Y-H, Yu C-H. Clinical effectiveness of laser acupuncture in the treatment of temporomandibular joint disorder. Journal of the Formosan Medical Association. 2014;113(8):535–539.

[45] Gottschling S, Meyer S, Gribova I, Distler L, Berrang J, Gortner L, et al. Laser acupuncture in children with headache: A double-blind, randomized, bicenter, placebo-controlled trial. Pain. 2008;137(2):405–412.

[46] Ip D, Fu N-Y. Two-year follow-up of low-level laser therapy for elderly with painful adhesive capsulitis of the shoulder. Journal of Pain Research. 2015;8:247–252.

[47] Hu W-L, Chang C-H, Hung Y-C. Clinical observations on laser acupuncture in simple obesity therapy. The American Journal of Chinese Medicine. 2010;38(05):861–867.

Chapter 4

Pain Management of Herpes Zoster

Hwa Young Jung and Hyun Jeong Park

Additional information is available at the end of the chapter

http://dx.doi.org/10.5772/62873

Abstract

Herpes zoster (HZ) is a disease triggered by the reactivation of latent varicella zoster virus (VZV) in spinal or cranial sensory ganglia, and is characterized by a painful vesicular eruption in the affected dermatome. Postherpetic neuralgia (PHN) is a chronic, neuropathic pain that can persist long beyond resolution of visible cutaneous manifestations which is often resistant to current analgesic treatments. The lifetime prevalence of herpes zoster is approximately 20–30% and about 9–34% of these patients develop PHN depending on its definition. Clinical experience has shown that PHN often develops in cases of inadequate initial pain management resulting in increased pain intensity. This review provides an overview of the treatment options for HZ and PHN, focusing on the therapeutic modalities of pain management. The primary objectives of management of HZ are to inhibit viral replication, relieve pain, and prevent associated complications, such as PHN. General treatments for acute HZ are combination of antiviral therapy with a short course of corticosteroids at the onset of the disease in conjunction with an effective control of acute pain, including nonsteroidal anti-inflammatory drugs, acetaminophen, opioids, and anticonvulsants such as gabapentin or pregabalin. Treatment of PHN is often resistant to the current pharmacologic methods. Therefore, a multimodal analgesic treatment regimen including topical lidocaine and capsaicin, systemic therapies, and the interventional treatments is necessary to alleviate pain and its effect on quality of life. As the incidence of HZ increases with age, the number of patients with HZ and PHN may increase in the future considering the gradual aging of the general population. Appropriate management of HZ can reduce the duration and intensity of pain from HZ, and prevent the development of PHN. In addition, prophylactic zoster vaccination can prevent or reduce the incidence of HZ and PHN. Further efforts are needed to minimize pain of the patients suffering from HZ and PHN as it affects the quality of life in the aspect of both physical and psychological impairments.

Keywords: Herpes zoster, post-herpetic neuralgia, pain control, treatment of herpes zoster, management of post-herpetic neuralgia

1. Introduction

Herpes zoster (HZ) is caused by reactivation of latent varicella zoster virus (VZV) in sensory dorsal root ganglion cells, and is characterized by a painful, unilateral vesicular skin eruption in the affected dermatome. The lifetime risk of HZ is approximately 15–30% [1–3]. The incidence of herpes zoster is 1.5–3.0 per 1000 person-years in all ages and 7–11 per 1000 person-years in persons over 60 years of age in European and North American, according to studies [1–9]. Classically, the skin eruption is preceded by one to several days of stabbing, episodic or continuous pain in the affected area, although the pain may develop simultaneously or even following the skin eruption. Herpes zoster-associated pain tends to resolve over time, but approximately 10–50% of herpes zoster patients develop post-herpetic neuralgia (PHN) that can persist several years beyond resolution of visible cutaneous eruptions. The frequency of PHN has been reported to be from 10% to 50% depending on its definition [10]. PHN is typically defined as persistent pain 90 days after the acute onset of HZ [3, 11, 12]. The incidence of PHN by this definition is 10–20% [3, 12]. In approximately 15% of patients with PHN, the pain persists for up to two years [13]. Mechanism to cause PHN follows a classic paradigm of other forms of neuropathic pain. Sensitization of nociceptors occurs after inflammation of dorsal root ganglia by reactivation of varicella zoster virus, leading to hyperexcitability of sensory neurons. The spontaneous discharge and lower activation thresholds provoke exaggerated responses to stimuli, resulting in allodynia and hyperalgesia. The loss of function or death of dorsal horn neurons, contributes to a connectional state of central nervous system nociceptive pathways, after anatomic deafferentation. The central sensitization is initially temporary, but may become permanent [14, 15]. Clinical experiences have shown that immunocompromised patients and elderly individuals are at an increased risk of PHN, and early initiation of antiviral treatment may reduce the incidence of PHN [16]. This review focuses on the practical overview of the treatment options available for management of patients with acute HZ and PHN.

2. Treatment of acute herpes zoster

The management of acute HZ aims to inhibit ongoing viral replication and alleviate pain. Treatment modalities for acute HZ include antiviral agents, analgesics, corticosteroids, and neural blockade.

2.1. Antiviral agents

Acute HZ is treated with antiviral agents such as acyclovir, famciclovir, and valacyclovir [17–20].

These antiviral agents are nucleoside analogues which are phosphorylated by viral thymidine kinase and cellular kinases to a triphosphate form that inhibits viral DNA polymerase, leading to a decrease of viral replication. Other types of antiviral agents such as foscarnet, vidarabine, and cidofovir are not dependent on viral phosphorylation and noncompetitively block viral DNA polymerase. In general, famciclovir and valaciclovir are accepted to have higher and more reliable levels of antiviral activity and bioavailability, although there is no systematic data proving superior efficacy of one antiviral agent over another. In addition, valacyclovir and famciclovir shows greater patient compliance than acyclovir with less frequent dosing [21]. The main benefits of administration of antiviral agents within 72 hours are to reduce the severity and duration of zoster-associated pain and the incidence of PHN [16]. Therefore, the use of antiviral agents is crucial in treatment of HZ, and should be prescribed for patients with HZ as soon as possible. In complicated cases, especially in ophthalmic zoster, disseminated zoster, or Ramsay Hunt syndrome, and in patients failing oral treatment, intravenous therapy should be considered. Many clinical trials suggest that antiviral agents should be started within 3 days of the cutaneous eruption [22–24]. In general, the recommended duration of systemic antiviral agents for uncomplicated HZ is a seven-day course [17]. However, there is no solid consensus about whether it is beneficial to extend the duration of the treatment for patients with new onset vesicles after the seventh day, or for patients with either neurologic or ocular complications [21]. In herpes zoster ophthalmicus, the ophthalmic division of the fifth cranial nerve is involved, and the antiviral treatment should always be prescribed even after 3 days of the disease onset [17]. In any case of ophthalmic herpes zoster, the patient should be seen by an ophthalmologist as soon as possible, especially when vesicles on the side and tip of the nose (Hutchinson's sign) are present. In cases with the immunosuppressed patients, antiviral therapy should always be started earlier because of the increased risk of herpes zoster complications. The same doses as in immunocompetent patients are used in immunosuppressed patients. The dosing regimen of the antiviral agents used in acute herpes zoster is summarized in **Table 1**. Meanwhile, the efficacy of topical antiviral agents for acute HZ had been shown to lack evidence [21].

Drug	Regimen	
	Immunocompetent patient	Immunocompromised patient
Famciclovir	PO 500 mg every 8 hour for 7 days	PO 500 mg every 8 hour for 7–10 days
Valaciclovir	PO 1000 mg every 8 hour for 7 days	PO 1000 mg every 8 hour for 7–10 days
Acyclovir	PO 800 mg 5 times a day for 7 days	PO 800 mg 5 times a day for 7–10 days or IV 10 mg/kg every 8 hour for 7–10 days

PO, per oral, IV, intravenous.

Table 1. Summary of antiviral agents for treatment of acute herpes zoster.

2.2. Pain control

Since pain is the most troublesome symptom of herpes zoster, adequate pain management is the mainstream of the treatment in conjunction with antiviral therapy. Most patients require additional analgesics, although antiviral treatment may reduce the acute pain from HZ. In addition, the effective relief of acute pain may reduce the risk of progression to PHN, because severe acute pain is a risk factor for PHN. Acetaminophen, nonsteroidal anti-inflammatory drugs (NSAIDs), and opioid analgesia may be used initially [25]. In patients experiencing insufficient pain relief with these agents, adjuvant analgesics such as antidepressants and anticonvulsants are shown to be effective to alleviate acute pain from HZ [24]. If parts of the pain of acute HZ may have inflammatory component, corticosteroids have been used during the acute episode of HZ. In clinical trials with selected older individuals, corticosteroids accelerate healing of the cutaneous lesion, improve quality-of-life measures, aid to return to routine activities, and reduce analgesic use. Systemic steroids starting at about 1 mg/kg/day for about 1 week, followed by 0.5 mg/kg/day for 1 week, and 0.25 mg/kg/day for another 1 week regimen is proven to be adequate to achieve these benefits [21]. If pain is refractory to formerly discussed medications, nerve block or referral to a pain specialist for sympathetic and epidural neural blockade can be performed.

3. Treatment of postherpetic neuralgia

PHN is difficult to treat and often resistant to the current pharmacologic therapies. A multimodal analgesic treatment approach should be performed achieving both the efficacy and the tolerability of the therapeutic regimen [26]. Currently, Food and Drug Administration (FDA)-approved therapies for the treatment of PHN are the transdermal lidocaine and capsaicin patches, gabapentin, and pregabalin. Therapies often use off-label or over-the-counter medications for PHN include tricyclic antidepressants (TCAs), selective serotonin reuptake inhibitors (SSRIs), opioids, antiepileptics, and nonsteroidal anti-inflammatory drugs (NSAIDs). The dosing regimen and adverse effects of treatment options for PHN are summarized in **Table 2**.

Treatment	Regimen	Adverse effects
Topical agent		
Topical lidocaine	Maximum of three 5% lidocaine patches for 12 hours a day	Itching, burning sensation or erythema on the application site
Topical capsaicin	0.025% or 0.075% capsaicin cream 8% capsaicin patch	
Anticonvulsants		
Gabapentin	Starting dose of 300 mg a day to maximum dose of 3600 mg a day	Somnolence, dizziness, peripheral edema
Pregabalin	Starting dose of 100–150 mg a day to maximum dose of 600 mg a day	
Tricyclic antidepressant (TCAs)		
Amitriptyline	Starting dose of 10 mg at night to maximum dose of 100 mg at night	Dry mouth, sedation, constipation, increased appetite, blurred vision, tinnitus, euphoria, urinary
Nortriptyline	Starting dose of 10–25 mg at night	

Treatment	Regimen	Adverse effects
	with maintenance dose of 30–75 mg a day in divided doses	retention
Desipramine	Starting dose of 10–25 mg a day to maximum dose of 150 mg a day	
Opioid analgesics		
Tramadol	Starting dose of 50 mg every 4–6 hour (100–400 mg a day)	
Morphine	PO controlled release morphine: Starting dose of 10 mg at night to maximum dose of 200 mg a day or divided dose of 10–30 mg every 12 hour IV morphine: Target dose of 0.3 mg/kg over 1 hour to maximum dose of 25 mg with cardiopulmonary monitoring	Nausea, vomiting, constipation, drowsiness, dizziness, mood change, disorientation, somnolence, headache, seizures
Oxycodone	PO controlled release oxycodone: Starting dose of 10 mg twice a day to maximum dose of 60 mg a day	
Methadone	Starting dose of 5 mg at night escalating dosage till dose-limiting side effects	

PO, per oral, IV, intravenous.

Table 2. Summary of treatment options for pain management of post-herpetic neuralgia.

3.1. Pharmacological treatment

3.1.1. Topical agent

Topical application of anesthetics and analgesics may reduce pain with convenient delivery of the pharmaceutical effect, improved patient adherence, and direct access to the target site leading to decreased risk for systemic side effects. For localized and relatively mild pain, topical agents may be a reasonable choice, especially in patients who cannot tolerate systemic therapy. Currently available topical therapies include lidocaine and capsaicin patches. In addition, in a small group of patients, topical application of a cannabinoid receptor agonist resulted in pain reduction by more than 80% [27, 28].

3.1.1.1. *Topical lidocaine*

Lidocaine relieves pain by reducing the ectopic activity of sensory nerves. The 5% lidocaine patch has been shown in controlled clinical trials to produce significant pain relief in patients with PHN and allodynia [29–32]. Often 7–10 days of treatment is required before efficacy is noted. It is easy to use and systemic toxicity is not considered a significant risk in adults. Side effects are usually limited to application site reaction, such as skin redness or rash, which may necessitate the discontinuation of treatment. Therefore, topical lidocaine is a good first-line treatment for elderly patients who have contraindications to systemic agents. The lidocaine patch contains 5% lidocaine base, adhesive, and other ingredients. In general, maximum of three patches are applied over the affected area for 12 hours a day. In addition, eutectic mixture of local anesthetics (EMLA) cream applied once a day on the affected skin with an occlusive dressing may perform as an adjuvant therapy [33].

3.1.1.2. *Topical capsaicin*

Capsaicin is an alkaloid derived from hot chili peppers and acts as a transient receptor potential cation channel, subfamily V, member 1 agonist that activates afferent nociceptor terminals [34–36]. Topical capsaicin has proven to effectively reduce pain than placebo in patients with both musculoskeletal and neuropathic pain [37, 38]. Topical capsaicin demonstrates analgesia via a counter-irritant mechanism in which the irritation of the affected area masks the pain sensation of the skin. Also, repeated use of capsaicin results in depletion of substance P and other neuropeptides from nociceptive fibers leading to desensitization of nociceptive terminals [39]. Adverse effects are often limited to local reaction such as itching, burning sensation, soreness, and erythema at the site of application, which may slowly disappear after continued use. The systemic absorption is minimal. Application of low concentration (0.025 and 0.075%) cream formulations for several weeks have shown efficacy in neuropathic pain. An 8% capsaicin patch is also available for use in patients with PHN and HIV neuropathic pain [40, 41]. A Cochrane review in 2009 analyzed six studies treating with either a capsaicin 0.075% cream or single application of 8% patch for chronic neuropathic pain. The authors concluded that both concentrations of capsaicin may relieve pain, but there were insufficient data to prove the degree of the benefit [42].

Although topical capsaicin monotherapy is generally not considered satisfactory for patients with chronic pain, it can be helpful as an adjuvant therapy.

3.1.2. *Systemic treatment*

PHN is typically difficult to treat due to both unsatisfactory pain relieving effects of pharmaceuticals and dose limitations related to intolerable side effects and drug-drug interactions.

Mainly, three classes of medication are used as standard therapies to manage PHN: anticonvulsants, antidepressants (TCAs), and opioid analgesics.

3.1.2.1. *Anticonvulsants*

Many anticonvulsants have been studied to treat chronic neuropathic pain disorders including trigeminal neuralgia and PHN. Gabapentin and pregabalin have been documented as safe and well tolerated anticonvulsant drugs helping to reduce zoster-associated pain. The mechanism of the analgesic action of gabapentin and pregabalin has not been fully described. Both gabapentin and pregabalin bind to the same receptor, $\alpha 2\delta$ subunits of voltage-gated calcium channels in the central nervous system. Since gabapentin and pregabalin are both eliminated from the systemic circulation primarily by renal excretion as unchanged drugs, the dosage of these drugs should be adjusted based on the renal function of the patients.

3.1.2.1.1. *Gabapentin*

Gabapentin has been shown to be superior in relieving pain in 41–43% of patients with PHN compared to 12–23% in patients receiving placebo [43, 44]. Gabapentin is absorbed slowly and reaches a peak level at 3–4 hours after administration. Gabapentin is initiated at 300 mg daily, escalating up to 3600 mg/day as needed for pain control. Pain relief occurs as early as one week after the initiation of the treatment. Frequent adverse effects of gabapentin are somnolence, dizziness, and peripheral edema. These adverse effects are usually short-lived, but they sometimes require dose adjustment [29, 43].

3.1.2.1.2. *Pregabalin*

Pregabalin is a potent gabapentinoid and structural analog of γ-aminobutyric acid (GABA). It is an ion channel modulator that has rapid analgesic, anticonvulsive, and anxiolytic effects. Pregabalin has been shown to relieve pain by more than 50% in 50% of patients with PHN compared to 20% in placebo groups [45, 46]. Dizziness, somnolence, and peripheral edema were also the most often reported adverse effects for pregabalin, although pregabalin usually has fewer dose-related adverse events than gabapentin because of the lower doses used [45–47]. Pregabalin has improved pharmacokinetics with better absorption and steadier blood levels and a faster onset of action than gabapentin. Therefore, titration of pregabalin to the therapeutic dose range is more rapid [47]. Pregabalin can be given in two divided doses per day, offering greater convenience than gabapentin [47, 48]. In general, the starting dose is 100–150 mg/day in divided doses escalating to 300 mg/day within one week, considering tolerability and effectiveness. Further up regulation of the dose up to 600 mg/day in 2–4 weeks may be considered for patients who experience unsatisfactory effect.

3.1.2.2. *Tricyclic antidepressant*

The TCAs work by blocking neuronal uptake of noradrenaline and serotonin, thereby potentiating inhibition of spinal neurons involved in nociceptive perception. Since the TCAs also block α-adrenergic receptors and sodium channels, they are known to be useful in PHN in which damaged primary afferent neurons develop adrenergic sensitivity and generate ectopic impulses closely related to sodium-channel blockade. In several randomized, controlled trials, the TCAs have been shown to relieve pain in 44–67% of elderly patients with PHN [26, 49–51].

The reported adverse effects of the TCAs include excessive sedation, cognitive impairment, dry mouth, constipation, sexual dysfunction, and orthostatic dizziness. The contraindications of the TCAs are patients with cardiovascular disease, glaucoma, and urinary retention. In addition, the patients with high risk of suicide are administered with caution. In general, the starting dose of TCAs is 10–25 mg/night for elderly patients. The dose may be increased by 25 mg nightly up to maximal dose. TCAs such as amitriptyline, nortriptyline, desipramine are well studied and documented as effective managements of PHN.

3.1.2.2.1. Amitriptyline

Amitriptyline is a tricyclic antidepressant that is widely used to treat various chronic neuropathic pains including PHN. However, there is insufficient evidence to recommend amitriptyline as a first-line agent for neuropathic pain with an overestimation of treatment effect. A Cochrane review in 2015 analyzed 17 studies involving 1342 oral amitriptyline-treated participants. The authors concluded that amitriptyline should continue to be used as part of the treatment of neuropathic pain, but only a minority of people will achieve satisfactory pain relief [52]. Amitriptyline is started at a low dose of 10 mg/night, with gradual dose increase up to 100 mg/night [11].

3.1.2.2.2. Nortriptyline

Nortriptyline, along with desipramine, is a preferred alternative treatment to amitriptyline because of its lesser adverse effects for the elderly such as cardiac problems, sedation, cognitive impairment, orthostatic hypotension, and constipation [53]. A recent Cochrane review in 2015 analyzed six studies treating 310 participants with various neuropathic pain conditions. The authors concluded that little evidence supports the use of nortriptyline as effective treatment for neuropathic pain [54]. The starting dose is 10–25 mg/night and the dosage may be increased by 25 mg/day with 1 week interval. In general, maintenance dose is 30–75 mg daily in divided doses, or a single night dose [11]. The most common side effects include dry mouth, sedation, constipation, increased appetite, mild blurred vision, tinnitus, and often euphoria and mania [55].

In a double-blind, randomized controlled trials, patients with diabetic polyneuropathy or PHN were randomized to receive nortriptyline and gabapentin, alone or in combination [56]. Combination regimen of gabapentin and nortriptyline produced greater pain relief than either agent alone. Therefore, combination therapy may benefit patients with PHN, but with higher risk of adverse effects than with either drug alone.

3.1.2.2.3. Desipramine

A Cochrane review in 2014 analyzed five studies treating 177 participants with painful diabetic neuropathy or PHN. The authors concluded that this review found little evidence to support the use of desipramine as effective treatment for neuropathic pain, although there was very low quality evidence of benefit and harm [57]. In randomized, placebo-controlled, double-blind, crossover studies, amitriptyline and desipramine have been shown to be effective for the treatment of PHN [58, 59]. Results from these studies showed that 67% of patients taking amitriptyline rated their pain relief as good to excellent, and 63% of patients taking desipramine rated their pain relief as moderate or better. Typically, the initial dose of desipramine for treatment of PHN is 10–25 mg/day with a maximum dose of 150 mg/day [11].

3.1.2.3. *Opioid analgesics*

Pain management with opioids may also alleviate PHN. Although effective in treating PHN, the issue of tolerance and concerns of misuse and abuse often tends to prevent opioids from being used as first-line agents. Opioids regulate pain binding to the opioid receptors such as μ, κ, δ and nociceptors present in both central and peripheral nervous system. The opioid receptors are activated by binding to inhibitory G-proteins, resulting in closure of voltage-gated calcium channels. This process leads to a cascade of potassium efflux causing hyperpolarization and reduced cyclic adenosine monophosphate level, hence decreasing the neuronal excitability. Additionally, opioids are capable of diverse and complex pharmacologic effects because they may function with various potencies acting as an agonist, partial agonist, or an antagonist binding to more than one receptor subtype. Side effects of opioids include constipation, cardiorespiratory dysfunction, sedation, nausea/vomiting, and histamine release [11]. Since constipation is a major side effect in elderly persons, bulk laxatives should be recommended. Additionally, the fact that many patients with PHN are elderly and have other underlying diseases for which they are taking medication emphasizes the need for close monitoring of adverse effects [11, 30, 60].

3.1.2.3.1. *Tramadol*

Tramadol is a synthetic 4-phenyl-piperidine analogue of codeine and acts as an analgesic with both opioid and non-opioid analgesic activity. Besides the opioid analgesic activity, it works via inhibition of noradrenaline reuptake and stimulation of serotonin release at the spinal level. Thus, it has properties of both an opioid and a TCA. In a randomized clinical trial, tramadol was proven to be an agent that significantly improve quality of life and alleviate pain in patients with PHN [61]. Adverse effects of tramadol include nausea, vomiting, constipation, drowsiness, dizziness, somnolence, headache, and seizures. Concomitant use of SSRIs, selective serotonin-and norepinephrine-reuptake inhibitor (SSNRIs), or TCAs should be avoided and drug interactions should be monitored [24]. It is generally dosed at 100–400 mg/day, in divided doses. The starting dose is 50 mg every 4–6 hours [26, 49].

3.1.2.3.2. *Morphine*

In a crossover trial with patients suffering PHN, both controlled release morphine and TCAs provided significant pain relief compared to placebo group [62]. In this report, patients preferred treatment with opioid analgesics to either TCAs or placebo, despite a higher incidence of adverse effects and more dropout patients during opioid treatment. In another crossover trial, patients with diabetic polyneuropathy or PHN were randomized to daily active placebo, sustained-release morphine, gabapentin, and a combination of gabapentin and morphine [63]. Combination regimen with morphine and gabapentin showed superior effect in pain relief than either agent alone or the active placebo, but with increased adverse effects. The starting dose of oral controlled release morphine is 10 mg/night and the dose is increased twice weekly till maximal dose of 200 mg/day. Also, it can be given at divided dose of 10–30 mg every 12 hours as needed [62]. For intravenous morphine, the target dose is 0.3 mg/kg over 1 hour, up to a maximum of 25 mg with cardiorespiratory monitoring in inpatient setting [64]. The adverse effects include nausea, vomiting, constipation, drowsiness, dizziness, mood change, and disorientation [26, 49].

3.1.2.3.3. Oxycodone

A Cochrane review in 2014 analyzed three studies treating 254 participants with painful diabetic neuropathy or PHN. In all three studies, controlled release oxycodone was used with doses titrated up to a maximum of 60–120 mg daily. The authors concluded that no convincing, unbiased evidence suggesting oxycodone is of value in treating patients with painful diabetic neuropathy or PHN exists [65]. However, other randomized, placebo-controlled crossover trials suggest greater efficacy of controlled release oxycodone over placebo [66]. The dose is 10 mg twice daily, up to a maximum of 60 mg/day. Adverse effects are typical of other opioids [30].

3.1.2.3.4. Methadone

Methadone is a synthetic opioid agonist that exhibits a potent antagonist effect on glutamate N-methyl-D-aspartate (NMDA) receptors. Although there is a great paucity of clinical evidence regarding the treatment effect of methadone on PHN, methadone may be tried as an adjunctive treatment for PHN. In a recent double blind and placebo controlled study, methadone, when compared to placebo, did not significantly affect the intensity of spontaneous pain, as measured by the visual analogue scale [67]. However, the intensity of spontaneous pain was significantly decreased after the methadone treatment, compared to placebo by the category verbal scale (50% improved after the methadone treatment, none after the placebo, $p=0.031$). Evoked pain was reduced under methadone compared to placebo (50% improved after the methadone treatment, none after the placebo, $p=0.031$). The starting dose is 5 mg/night and is increased till maximal pain relief is achieved or occurrence of dose-limiting side effects. Methadone has a high intestinal absorption, and most of the drug is excreted in feces with no significant renal elimination, hence this drug is safe for patients with renal failure [68].

3.2. Non-pharmacological treatment

As a general rule, non-pharmacological, interventional pain management is frequently used in acute settings or in patients who have failed the standard therapies.

3.2.1. *Nerve block*

The interventional treatments including sublesional anesthesia, epidural blocks, intrathecal injection, and sympathetic nerve blocks with and without corticosteroids have been reported in large series, but rarely studied in a controlled manner. They have limited evidence of effective treatment of PHN [29]. Epidural block with local anesthetics and steroids is not effective in providing long-term pain relief in patients with PHN. Sympathetic nerve blocks have shown beneficial effects in patients with acute HZ, but with insufficient effect in providing long-term pain alleviation in patients with PHN [69]. Long-term pain relief by peripheral nerve block using local anesthetics has been reported, but with limited quality of the evidence [70].

3.2.2. *Spinal cord stimulation*

Spinal cord stimulation (SCS) has been used for the management of chronic neuropathic pain disorders [71, 72]. However, no randomized controlled study supports the usefulness of SCS. Studies on SCS were all case series with a small number of cases [73–75]. Therefore, SCS should be used only as a next resort after intrathecal steroid injections or nerve blocks in patient's refractory to pharmacological treatments of PHN.

3.2.3. *Transcutaneous electrical nerve stimulation*

Transcutaneous electrical nerve stimulation (TENS) is the use of electric current produced by a device to stimulate the nerves at a strong but nonpainful intensity that can produce pain relief [76]. TENS is an adjunctive therapy that has shown efficacy in transiently relieving neuropathic pain [77, 78]. In a study of TENS for patients with chronic pain, approximately 30% of patients with PHN fail to respond to TENS and among patients who respond initially, only a third continue to obtain pain relief after 2 years [77]. In a recent pilot randomized study of patients who were refractory to previous pharmacological therapy, the patients were treated with TENS with a biofeedback capability [79]. After every two treatments with the sham and true device, the patients were required to fill out a standard neuropathic pain scale score. The patients had choices to select the other device after three consecutive treatments if they felt an insufficient relief in their pain. The true device was chosen over the sham device by all patients. The majority of these patients treated by the true device reported a significant decrease in pain scores.

3.2.4. *Botulinum toxin*

BTX-A may play an adjunctive role as a promising therapeutic modality for PHN with its proven efficacy, safety, and tolerability. Botulinum toxin A (BTX-A) blocks acetylcholine by cleaving synaptosomal-associated protein of 25 kDa (SNAP25), which participates in the formation of the exocytic soluble N-ethylmaleimide–sensitive factor attachment protein receptor complex(SNARE) that is essential for the fusion of acetylocholine-containing vesicles with the presynaptic membrane [80, 81]. Therefore, the local peripheral BTX-A injection may result in anti-nociceptive effect associated with the inhibition of formalin-induced glutamate release, substance P and calcitonin gene–related peptide, which participates in the neurogenic inflammation [82]. There are several case series and randomized controlled trials supporting both therapeutic benefit and safety of BTX-A on PHN patients [83–88]. In these studies, no significant safety issues including local or systemic adverse effects was raised except the pain during injections. A possible consideration to BTX-A use is that, unlike other therapeutic modalities for PHN, it may induce antitoxin antibodies that could probably limit the long-term repetitive use of the treatment [89].

4. Vaccination against herpes zoster

In a randomized trial with elderly patients, adult vaccination reduced the incidence of herpes zoster by 51% and the incidence of postherpetic neuralgia by 66%. In patients 70 years of age or older as compared with patients 60 to 69 years of age, the vaccine was less effective in reducing the risk of herpes zoster (38% reduction) but demonstrated similar protection against PHN (67% reduction) [90]. A live attenuated VZV vaccine has been available since 2006. It is a one-dose, high-potency vaccine originally approved for immunocompetent persons 60 years of age or older, but in 2011, it was approved to include persons aged 50–59 years [91]. This live attenuated vaccine is contraindicated in pregnant women and immunocompromised individuals. The reported side effects of the vaccine are minor, such as erythema, pain, and an itching sensation at the injection site, and fever [90]. Regarding the persistence of vaccine efficacy, the Shingles Prevention Study demonstrated the proven efficacy of the vaccine through four years post-vaccination. Additionally, the Short-Term Persistence Substudy subsequently demonstrated the persistence of vaccine efficacy through five years post-vaccination, although the efficacy beyond five years is uncertain [92]. Overall, the zoster vaccination can be used as the first line management for the prevention of HZ and PHN.

5. Conclusion

As the general population ages, the number of patients suffering from HZ and PHN may increase gradually in the future. Diverse and comprehensive efforts are necessary as patients suffering from acute HZ and PHN are burdened by a worse quality of life due to both physical and psychological impairments [11]. We summarized the management of acute HZ and PHN to shorten the duration and intensity of pain. In order to choose the optimal treatment, clinicians should consider issues related to efficacy, safety, and tolerability in conjunction with individuals' goals of therapy, preferences, and adherence issues. Finally, regardless of the agents chosen, the adverse effects and drug interactions should always be considered to provide safe and effective management of pain.

http://dx.doi.org/10.5772/62873

Acknowledgements

This work was supported by the Basic Science Research program through the National Research Foundation of Korea (NRF), which is funded by the Ministry of Education, Science and Technology (2015R1C1A2A01055073).

Author details

Hwa Young Jung and Hyun Jeong Park*

*Address all correspondence to: hjpark@catholic.ac.kr

Department of Dermatology, College of Medicine, The Catholic University of Korea, Seoul, Republic of Korea

Reference

[1] Insinga RP, Itzler RF, Pellissier JM, Saddier P, Nikas AA. The incidence of herpes zoster in a United States administrative database. Journal of General Internal Medicine. 2005;20(8):748–53.

[2] Vazquez M, Shapiro ED. Varicella vaccine and infection with varicella-zoster virus. The New England Journal of Medicine. 2005;352(5):439–40.

[3] Yawn BP, Saddier P, Wollan PC, St Sauver JL, Kurland MJ, Sy LS. A population-based study of the incidence and complication rates of herpes zoster before zoster vaccine introduction. Mayo Clinic Proceedings. 2007;82(11):1341–9.

[4] Donahue JG, Choo PW, Manson JE, Platt R. The incidence of herpes zoster. Archives of Internal Medicine. 1995;155(15):1605–9.

[5] Gauthier A, Breuer J, Carrington D, Martin M, Remy V. Epidemiology and cost of herpes zoster and post-herpetic neuralgia in the United Kingdom. Epidemiology and Infection. 2009;137(1):38–47.

[6] Mullooly JP, Riedlinger K, Chun C, Weinmann S, Houston H. Incidence of herpes zoster, 1997–2002. Epidemiology and Infection. 2005;133(2):245–53.

[7] Schmader K, George LK, Burchett BM, Pieper CF, Hamilton JD. Racial differences in the occurrence of herpes zoster. The Journal of Infectious Diseases. 1995;171(3):701–4.

[8] Schmader K, Gnann JW, Jr., Watson CP. The epidemiological, clinical, and pathological rationale for the herpes zoster vaccine. The Journal of Infectious Diseases. 2008;197 Suppl 2:S207-15.

[9] Thomas SL, Hall AJ. What does epidemiology tell us about risk factors for herpes zoster? The Lancet Infectious Diseases. 2004;4(1):26–33.

[10] Cohen JI. Clinical practice: Herpes zoster. The New England Journal of Medicine. 2013;369(3):255–63.

[11] Johnson RW, Rice AS. Clinical practice. Postherpetic neuralgia. The New England Journal of Medicine. 2014;371(16):1526–33.

[12] Arvin A. Aging, immunity, and the varicella-zoster virus. The New England Journal of Medicine. 2005;352(22):2266–7.

[13] Zin CS, Nissen LM, Smith MT, O'Callaghan JP, Moore BJ. An update on the pharmacological management of post-herpetic neuralgia and painful diabetic neuropathy. CNS Drugs. 2008;22(5):417–42.

[14] Bennett GJ. Hypotheses on the pathogenesis of herpes zoster-associated pain. Annals of Neurology. 1994;35 Suppl:S38–41.

[15] Cervero F, Laird JM. Mechanisms of touch-evoked pain (allodynia): a new model. Pain. 1996;68(1):13–23.

[16] Panlilio LM, Christo PJ, Raja SN. Current management of postherpetic neuralgia. The Neurologist. 2002;8(6):339–50.

[17] Bruxelle J, Pinchinat S. Effectiveness of antiviral treatment on acute phase of herpes zoster and development of post herpetic neuralgia: review of international publications. Medecine et Maladies Infectieuses. 2012;42(2):53–8.

[18] Jackson JL, Gibbons R, Meyer G, Inouye L. The effect of treating herpes zoster with oral acyclovir in preventing postherpetic neuralgia. A meta-analysis. Archives of Internal Medicine. 1997;157(8):909–12.

[19] Tyring S, Barbarash RA, Nahlik JE, Cunningham A, Marley J, Heng M, et al. Famciclovir for the treatment of acute herpes zoster: effects on acute disease and postherpetic neuralgia. A randomized, double-blind, placebo-controlled trial. Collaborative Famciclovir Herpes Zoster Study Group. Annals of Internal Medicine. 1995;123(2):89–96.

[20] Beutner KR, Friedman DJ, Forszpaniak C, Andersen PL, Wood MJ. Valaciclovir compared with acyclovir for improved therapy for herpes zoster in immunocompetent adults. Antimicrobial Agents and Chemotherapy. 1995;39(7):1546–53.

[21] Dworkin RH, Johnson RW, Breuer J, Gnann JW, Levin MJ, Backonja M, et al. Recommendations for the management of herpes zoster. Clinical Infectious Diseases: An Official Publication of the Infectious Diseases Society of America. 2007;44 Suppl 1:S1–26.

[22] Shafran SD, Tyring SK, Ashton R, Decroix J, Forszpaniak C, Wade A, et al. Once, twice, or three times daily famciclovir compared with aciclovir for the oral treatment of herpes

zoster in immunocompetent adults: a randomized, multicenter, double-blind clinical trial. Journal of Clinical Virology: The Official Publication of the Pan American Society for Clinical Virology. 2004;29(4):248–53.

[23] Shen MC, Lin HH, Lee SS, Chen YS, Chiang PC, Liu YC. Double-blind, randomized, acyclovir-controlled, parallel-group trial comparing the safety and efficacy of famciclovir and acyclovir in patients with uncomplicated herpes zoster. Journal of Microbiology, Immunology, and Infection = Wei mian yu gan ran za zhi. 2004;37(2):75–81.

[24] Sampathkumar P, Drage LA, Martin DP. Herpes zoster (shingles) and postherpetic neuralgia. Mayo Clinic Proceedings. 2009;84(3):274–80.

[25] Dworkin RH, Barbano RL, Tyring SK, Betts RF, McDermott MP, Pennella-Vaughan J, et al. A randomized, placebo-controlled trial of oxycodone and of gabapentin for acute pain in herpes zoster. Pain. 2009;142(3):209–17.

[26] Hempenstall K, Nurmikko TJ, Johnson RW, A'Hern RP, Rice AS. Analgesic therapy in postherpetic neuralgia: a quantitative systematic review. PLoS Medicine. 2005;2(7):e164.

[27] Beiteke U, Bigge S, Reichenberger C, Gralow I. Pain and pain management in dermatology. Journal der Deutschen Dermatologischen Gesellschaft = Journal of the German Society of Dermatology: JDDG. 2015;13(10):967–87.

[28] Phan NQ, Siepmann D, Gralow I, Stander S. Adjuvant topical therapy with a cannabinoid receptor agonist in facial postherpetic neuralgia. Journal der Deutschen Dermatologischen Gesellschaft = Journal of the German Society of Dermatology: JDDG. 2010;8(2):88–91.

[29] Jeon YH. Herpes Zoster and Postherpetic Neuralgia: Practical Consideration for Prevention and Treatment. The Korean Journal of Pain. 2015;28(3):177–84.

[30] Gan EY, Tian EA, Tey HL. Management of herpes zoster and post-herpetic neuralgia. American Journal of Clinical Dermatology. 2013;14(2):77–85.

[31] Rowbotham MC, Davies PS, Verkempinck C, Galer BS. Lidocaine patch: double-blind controlled study of a new treatment method for post-herpetic neuralgia. Pain. 1996;65(1):39–44.

[32] Galer BS, Jensen MP, Ma T, Davies PS, Rowbotham MC. The lidocaine patch 5% effectively treats all neuropathic pain qualities: results of a randomized, double-blind, vehicle-controlled, 3-week efficacy study with use of the neuropathic pain scale. The Clinical Journal of Pain. 2002;18(5):297–301.

[33] Galer BS, Rowbotham MC, Perander J, Friedman E. Topical lidocaine patch relieves postherpetic neuralgia more effectively than a vehicle topical patch: results of an enriched enrollment study. Pain. 1999;80(3):533–8.

[34] Enamandram M, Rathmell JP, Kimball AB. Chronic pain management in dermatology: a guide to assessment and nonopioid pharmacotherapy. Journal of the American Academy of Dermatology. 2015;73(4):563–73; quiz 73–4.

[35] Irving GA, Backonja MM, Dunteman E, Blonsky ER, Vanhove GF, Lu SP, et al. A multicenter, randomized, double-blind, controlled study of NGX-4010, a high-concentration capsaicin patch, for the treatment of postherpetic neuralgia. Pain Medicine (Malden, Mass). 2011;12(1):99–109.

[36] Derry S, Sven-Rice A, Cole P, Tan T, Moore RA. Topical capsaicin (high concentration) for chronic neuropathic pain in adults. The Cochrane Database of Systematic Reviews. 2013;2:Cd007393.

[37] Mason L, Moore RA, Derry S, Edwards JE, McQuay HJ. Systematic review of topical capsaicin for the treatment of chronic pain. BMJ (Clinical research ed). 2004;328(7446): 991.

[38] Casanueva B, Rodero B, Quintial C, Llorca J, Gonzalez-Gay MA. Short-term efficacy of topical capsaicin therapy in severely affected fibromyalgia patients. Rheumatology International. 2013;33(10):2665–70.

[39] Watson CP, Tyler KL, Bickers DR, Millikan LE, Smith S, Coleman E. A randomized vehicle-controlled trial of topical capsaicin in the treatment of postherpetic neuralgia. Clinical Therapeutics. 1993;15(3):510–26.

[40] Sawynok J. Topical and peripherally acting analgesics. Pharmacological Reviews. 2003;55(1):1–20.

[41] Zhang WY, Li Wan Po A. The effectiveness of topically applied capsaicin. A meta-analysis. European Journal of Clinical Pharmacology. 1994;46(6):517–22.

[42] Derry S, Lloyd R, Moore RA, McQuay HJ. Topical capsaicin for chronic neuropathic pain in adults. The Cochrane Database of Systematic Reviews. 2009(4):Cd007393.

[43] Rowbotham M, Harden N, Stacey B, Bernstein P, Magnus-Miller L. Gabapentin for the treatment of postherpetic neuralgia: a randomized controlled trial. Jama. 1998;280(21): 1837–42.

[44] Rice AS, Maton S. Gabapentin in postherpetic neuralgia: a randomised, double blind, placebo controlled study. Pain. 2001;94(2):215–24.

[45] Dworkin RH, Corbin AE, Young JP, Jr., Sharma U, LaMoreaux L, Bockbrader H, et al. Pregabalin for the treatment of postherpetic neuralgia: a randomized, placebo-controlled trial. Neurology. 2003;60(8):1274–83.

[46] Moore RA, Straube S, Wiffen PJ, Derry S, McQuay HJ. Pregabalin for acute and chronic pain in adults. The Cochrane Database of Systematic Reviews. 2009(3):Cd007076.

[47] Sabatowski R, Galvez R, Cherry DA, Jacquot F, Vincent E, Maisonobe P, et al. Pregabalin reduces pain and improves sleep and mood disturbances in patients with post-herpetic

neuralgia: results of a randomised, placebo-controlled clinical trial. Pain. 2004;109(1–2):26–35.

[48] Christo PJ, Hobelmann G, Maine DN. Post-herpetic neuralgia in older adults: evidence-based approaches to clinical management. Drugs & Aging. 2007;24(1):1–19.

[49] Dworkin RH, O'Connor AB, Backonja M, Farrar JT, Finnerup NB, Jensen TS, et al. Pharmacologic management of neuropathic pain: evidence-based recommendations. Pain. 2007;132(3):237–51.

[50] Dubinsky RM, Kabbani H, El-Chami Z, Boutwell C, Ali H. Practice parameter: treatment of postherpetic neuralgia: an evidence-based report of the Quality Standards Subcommittee of the American Academy of Neurology. Neurology. 2004;63(6):959–65.

[51] Saarto T, Wiffen PJ. Antidepressants for neuropathic pain: a Cochrane review. Journal of Neurology, Neurosurgery, and Psychiatry. 2010;81(12):1372–3.

[52] Moore RA, Derry S, Aldington D, Cole P, Wiffen PJ. Amitriptyline for neuropathic pain in adults. The Cochrane Database of Systematic Reviews. 2015;7:Cd008242.

[53] Watson CP, Vernich L, Chipman M, Reed K. Nortriptyline versus amitriptyline in postherpetic neuralgia: a randomized trial. Neurology. 1998;51(4):1166–71.

[54] Derry S, Wiffen PJ, Aldington D, Moore RA. Nortriptyline for neuropathic pain in adults. The Cochrane Database of Systematic Reviews. 2015;1:Cd011209.

[55] Liu WQ, Kanungo A, Toth C. Equivalency of tricyclic antidepressants in open-label neuropathic pain study. Acta Neurologica Scandinavica. 2014;129(2):132–41.

[56] Gilron I, Bailey JM, Tu D, Holden RR, Jackson AC, Houlden RL. Nortriptyline and gabapentin, alone and in combination for neuropathic pain: a double-blind, randomised controlled crossover trial. Lancet (London, England). 2009;374(9697):1252–61.

[57] Hearn L, Moore RA, Derry S, Wiffen PJ, Phillips T. Desipramine for neuropathic pain in adults. The Cochrane Database of Systematic Reviews. 2014;9:Cd011003.

[58] Watson CP, Evans RJ, Reed K, Merskey H, Goldsmith L, Warsh J. Amitriptyline versus placebo in postherpetic neuralgia. Neurology. 1982;32(6):671–3.

[59] Kishore-Kumar R, Max MB, Schafer SC, Gaughan AM, Smoller B, Gracely RH, et al. Desipramine relieves postherpetic neuralgia. Clinical Pharmacology and Therapeutics. 1990;47(3):305–12.

[60] Khadem T, Stevens V. Therapeutic options for the treatment of postherpetic neuralgia: a systematic review. Journal of Pain & Palliative Care Pharmacotherapy. 2013;27(3): 268–83.

[61] Boureau F, Legallicier P, Kabir-Ahmadi M. Tramadol in post-herpetic neuralgia: a randomized, double-blind, placebo-controlled trial. Pain. 2003;104(1–2):323–31.

[62] Raja SN, Haythornthwaite JA, Pappagallo M, Clark MR, Travison TG, Sabeen S, et al. Opioids versus antidepressants in postherpetic neuralgia: a randomized, placebo-controlled trial. Neurology. 2002;59(7):1015–21.

[63] Gilron I, Bailey JM, Tu D, Holden RR, Weaver DF, Houlden RL. Morphine, gabapentin, or their combination for neuropathic pain. The New England Journal of Medicine. 2005;352(13):1324–34.

[64] Rowbotham MC, Reisner-Keller LA, Fields HL. Both intravenous lidocaine and morphine reduce the pain of postherpetic neuralgia. Neurology. 1991;41(7):1024–8.

[65] Gaskell H, Moore RA, Derry S, Stannard C. Oxycodone for neuropathic pain and fibromyalgia in adults. The Cochrane Database of Systematic Reviews. 2014;6:Cd010692.

[66] Watson CP, Babul N. Efficacy of oxycodone in neuropathic pain: a randomized trial in postherpetic neuralgia. Neurology. 1998;50(6):1837–41.

[67] Teixeira MJ, Okada M, Moscoso AS, Puerta MY, Yeng LT, Galhardoni R, et al. Methadone in post-herpetic neuralgia: A pilot proof-of-concept study. Clinics (Sao Paulo, Brazil). 2013;68(7):1057–60.

[68] Bruera E, Palmer JL, Bosnjak S, Rico MA, Moyano J, Sweeney C, et al. Methadone versus morphine as a first-line strong opioid for cancer pain: a randomized, double-blind study. Journal of Clinical Oncology: Official Journal of the American Society of Clinical Oncology. 2004;22(1):185–92.

[69] Kumar V, Krone K, Mathieu A. Neuraxial and sympathetic blocks in herpes zoster and postherpetic neuralgia: an appraisal of current evidence. Regional Anesthesia and Pain Medicine. 2004;29(5):454–61.

[70] Doi K, Nikai T, Sakura S, Saito Y. Intercostal nerve block with 5% tetracaine for chronic pain syndromes. Journal of Clinical Anesthesia. 2002;14(1):39–41.

[71] Moriyama K. Effect of temporary spinal cord stimulation on postherpetic neuralgia in the thoracic nerve area. Neuromodulation: Journal of the International Neuromodulation Society. 2009;12(1):39–43.

[72] Benzon HT, Chekka K, Darnule A, Chung B, Wille O, Malik K. Evidence-based case report: the prevention and management of postherpetic neuralgia with emphasis on interventional procedures. Regional Anesthesia and Pain Medicine. 2009;34(5):514–21.

[73] Meglio M, Cioni B, Prezioso A, Talamonti G. Spinal cord stimulation (SCS) in the treatment of postherpetic pain. Acta Neurochirurgica Supplementum. 1989;46:65–6.

[74] Sanchez-Ledesma MJ, Garcia-March G, Diaz-Cascajo P, Gomez-Moreta J, Broseta J. Spinal cord stimulation in deafferentation pain. Stereotactic and Functional Neurosurgery. 1989;53(1):40–5.

[75] Kumar K, Hunter G, Demeria D. Spinal cord stimulation in treatment of chronic benign pain: challenges in treatment planning and present status, a 22-year experience. Neurosurgery. 2006;58(3):481–96; discussion–96.

[76] Xu G, Xu G, Feng Y, Tang WZ, Lv ZW. Transcutaneous electrical nerve stimulation in combination with cobalamin injection for postherpetic neuralgia: a single-center randomized controlled trial. American Journal of Physical Medicine & Rehabilitation / Association of Academic Physiatrists. 2014;93(4):287–98.

[77] Bates JA, Nathan PW. Transcutaneous electrical nerve stimulation for chronic pain. Anaesthesia. 1980;35(8):817–22.

[78] Barbarisi M, Pace MC, Passavanti MB, Maisto M, Mazzariello L, Pota V, et al. Pregabalin and transcutaneous electrical nerve stimulation for postherpetic neuralgia treatment. The Clinical Journal of Pain. 2010;26(7):567–72.

[79] Ing MR, Hellreich PD, Johnson DW, Chen JJ. Transcutaneous electrical nerve stimulation for chronic post-herpetic neuralgia. International journal of dermatology. 2015;54(4):476–80.

[80] Blasi J, Chapman ER, Link E, Binz T, Yamasaki S, De Camilli P, et al. Botulinum neurotoxin A selectively cleaves the synaptic protein SNAP-25. Nature. 1993;365(6442): 160–3.

[81] Hay JC. SNARE complex structure and function. Experimental Cell Research. 2001;271(1):10–21.

[82] Cui M, Khanijou S, Rubino J, Aoki KR. Subcutaneous administration of botulinum toxin A reduces formalin-induced pain. Pain. 2004;107(1–2):125–33.

[83] Apalla Z, Sotiriou E, Lallas A, Lazaridou E, Ioannides D. Botulinum toxin A in postherpetic neuralgia: a parallel, randomized, double-blind, single-dose, placebo-controlled trial. The Clinical Journal of Pain. 2013;29(10):857–64.

[84] Sotiriou E, Apalla Z, Panagiotidou D, Ioannidis D. Severe post-herpetic neuralgia successfully treated with botulinum toxin A: three case reports. Acta Dermato-venereologica. 2009;89(2):214–5.

[85] Liu HT, Tsai SK, Kao MC, Hu JS. Botulinum toxin A relieved neuropathic pain in a case of post-herpetic neuralgia. Pain Medicine (Malden, Mass). 2006;7(1):89–91.

[86] Ranoux D, Attal N, Morain F, Bouhassira D. Botulinum toxin type A induces direct analgesic effects in chronic neuropathic pain. Annals of Neurology. 2008;64(3):274–83.

[87] Yuan RY, Sheu JJ, Yu JM, Chen WT, Tseng IJ, Chang HH, et al. Botulinum toxin for diabetic neuropathic pain: a randomized double-blind crossover trial. Neurology. 2009;72(17):1473–8.

[88] Xiao L, Mackey S, Hui H, Xong D, Zhang Q, Zhang D. Subcutaneous injection of botulinum toxin a is beneficial in postherpetic neuralgia. Pain Medicine (Malden, Mass). 2010;11(12):1827–33.

[89] Naumann M, Carruthers A, Carruthers J, Aurora SK, Zafonte R, Abu-Shakra S, et al. Meta-analysis of neutralizing antibody conversion with onabotulinumtoxinA (BOTOX(R)) across multiple indications. Movement Disorders: Official Journal of the Movement Disorder Society. 2010;25(13):2211–8.

[90] Oxman MN, Levin MJ, Johnson GR, Schmader KE, Straus SE, Gelb LD, et al. A vaccine to prevent herpes zoster and postherpetic neuralgia in older adults. The New England Journal of Medicine. 2005;352(22):2271–84.

[91] Voelker R. FDA expands age range for shingles vaccine. Jama. 2011;305(15):1526.

[92] Schmader KE, Oxman MN, Levin MJ, Johnson G, Zhang JH, Betts R, et al. Persistence of the efficacy of zoster vaccine in the shingles prevention study and the short-term persistence substudy. Clinical Infectious Diseases: An Official Publication of the Infectious Diseases Society of America. 2012;55(10):1320–8.

Chapter 5

Pain Management in Knee Osteoarthritis

Shahnawaz Anwer and Ahmad Alghadir

Additional information is available at the end of the chapter

http://dx.doi.org/10.5772/62862

Abstract

Osteoarthritis (OA) of the knee is the commonest degenerative joint disease affecting older adults. Risk factors for the knee OA includes female gender, advanced age, overweight, obesity, previous knee injuries, previous knee surgery, and certain jobs that require continuous knee bending. Pain is the major symptom of knee OA and increased pain causes reduced physical function and poor quality of life. In addition to pain, patients may have joint stiffness, knee extensor muscle weakness, and altered proprioception. A multitude of structural, physical, and psychosocial factors influences symptom and severity of pain in knee OA. Rehabilitation of knee OA aims to train the patients in coping strategies, improves physical health, quality of life, and maintains their independence in daily livings. Management of knee OA often requires a combination of pharmacologic and nonpharmacologic treatment approaches.

Keywords: Knee, osteoarthritis, pain, rehabilitation, physiotherapy

1. Introduction

Osteoarthritis (OA) of the knee is a prevalent musculoskeletal disorder causing pain and disability in older population [1]. Worldwide statistics indicates more than 100 million individuals globally affected by OA [2, 3]. The prevalence of OA is expected to double at the end of the year 2020 [4]. The prevalence of symptomatic knee OA in male and female is approximately 40 and 47%, respectively [5]. Evidence of radiographic knee OA in the United States is approximately 19% in adults aged 45 years and older [5]. While male and female are equally affected by OA, it is reported to be more common in young adult male (<45 years) and in the older adult female (>45 years) [6–9].

Risk factors for the knee OA includes female gender, advanced age, overweight, obesity, previous knee injuries, previous knee surgery, and certain jobs that require continuous knee bending (kneeling and lifting) [10, 11]. Biomechanical factors including, abnormal joint congruity, muscle weakness, mal-alignment, or internal derangement of knee, facilitate the progression of knee OA in those persons, who are susceptible to the development of the knee OA [12, 13]. Lower extremity muscle weakness has vital role in the progression of the knee OA [14, 15]. Previous studies indicate that weaker quadriceps muscle is associated with symptomatic knee OA and weakness of muscles increases the risk of physical disability [14, 15].

Knee OA can be classified either symptomatically or radiographically. The Kellgren–Lawrence (KL) [16] grading scale has been used to diagnose radiographic knee OA. The symptomatic knee OA has been diagnosed clinically followed by radiographic confirmation.

The symptoms of knee OA includes pain, stiffness, limited range of motion, swelling, crepitus, and muscle weakness [17, 18]. Knee pain significantly influences physical function depending on the site of pain and unilateral or bilateral involvement [19]. Knee pain affects variety of activities including the limited ability to use stairs, standing up from the chair, walking on uneven terrain, floor sitting, and squatting [20–22].

Rehabilitation of knee OA aims to train the patients in coping strategies, improves physical health, quality of life, and maintains their independence in daily livings. These goals can be achieved by variety of interventions including, pharmacological approach, physical therapy, education, weight reduction, orthotic, and surgery.

2. Risk factors

There are variety of risk factors including age, gender, occupation, osteoporosis, genetics, nutritional factors, previous injury, knee extensor muscle weakness, and obesity [23, 24]. A recent meta-analysis provides further evidence that increased body mass index (BMI), past knee injury, age, female gender, and hand OA are the major risk factors causing knee OA [11]. The frequency of OA is increased in older population. In the United Kingdom, up to 40% people above the age of 65 years has been suffering from the symptoms associated with knee or hip OA [25]. While male and female are equally affected by OA, it is reported to be more common in the young adult male (<45 years) and in the older adult female (>45 years) [6–9].

A previous study reported some occupational activities, for example, kneeling, high levels of physical activity, farming, and construction work are potential risk factors for developing knee OA [11]. Another study reported double the risk of developing knee OA in individuals whose jobs required carrying and kneeling, or squatting activities compared to individuals whose jobs did not require such physical activities [26]. In addition, jobs which require repetitive task or sports, particularly endurance sports in which joint injuries are common, may predispose OA [27].

Obesity is recognized as major risk factors for mechanical joint damage, particularly in weight-bearing joints, and is often present with sedentary people with knee OA [28, 29]. The risk of incidence and progression of lower extremity OA increases with obesity [30], and the risk of knee OA increases four times more compared with individuals with a BMI of <30 kg/m^2 [31].

Another study reported 83% of the female participants had knee OA who were obese compared to 42% of non-obese control group [32]. In addition, obesity can alter the mechanics of joint and develop inflammation and cause increased pain [33, 34]. Furthermore, increased fat around the quadriceps muscle causes reduced activity of the muscle, resulting in decreased function [35].

Previous studies had reported knee extensor muscle weakness, a major risk factor for knee OA, especially in women [36, 37]. Other studies found knee extensor muscle weakness in people with knee OA compared to control subjects [7, 15, 38]. In addition, Segal et al. [39] reported low risk of symptomatic knee OA in individuals with greater quadriceps muscle strength. The weakness of quadriceps muscle causes reduced functional disability in knee OA [22]. Furthermore, the presence of pain causes disused atrophy which results quadriceps weakness in knee OA [14].

3. Diagnosis of osteoarthritis

The diagnosis of the OA often made clinically, and radiological features confirm the diagnosis. The presence of pain in the knee, morning stiffness lasting over the 30 min, limited movement, crepitus, swelling, and advanced age usually the main characteristics that indicate the diagnosis of knee OA. The narrowing of joint space, sclerosis of subchondral bone, and formation of subchondral cyst and osteophytes are radiological features seen in knee OA [40].

Kellgren and Lawrence [16] have developed a radiological scale to classify knee OA into four grades on antero-posterior view of radiograph taken in standing position. "Grade 0 is defined as no radiographic findings of osteoarthritis, Grade 1 as minute osteophytes of doubtful clinical significance, Grade 2 as definite osteophytes with unimpaired joint space, Grade 3 as definite osteophytes with moderate joint space narrowing, and Grade 4 as definite osteophytes with severe joint space narrowing and subchondral sclerosis" [41]. In addition, the American Rheumatism Association (ARA) has developed a more specific classification system in 1986, known as the American College of Rheumatology (ACR) criteria. These criteria included several validated clinical and radiological features [42].

4. Clinical manifestations

Pain is the major symptom of knee OA, and increased pain causes reduced physical function and poor quality of life [43]. In addition, knee pain causes difficulty in performing activities of daily livings including shopping, household chores, stair climbing as well as participation in social and outdoor activities [44]. Furthermore, pain related to knee OA influences work productivity and employment status [45]. In addition to pain, patients may have joint stiffness, knee extensor muscle weakness, and altered proprioception [46–48]. These symptoms often cause restriction in the ability to get up from the chair, difficulty in walking, and stair climbing [46]. Limping gait, poor limb alignment, and instability are some other features seen in people with knee OA [49]. A crepitus sound can be heard during movements due to the presence of irregular joint surfaces in knee OA [50].

A multitude of structural, physical, and psychosocial factors influences symptom and severity of pain in knee OA [43, 51, 52]. Although the role of nociceptors in the capsule, subchondral bone, ligaments, and other joint tissues precipitation symptom of pain was established, however, structural deformation in knee OA is not associated with the severity of pain [53]. Previous studies reported that the impairments in the physical and psychological functions are the major predictors of the severity of knee pain. Reduced muscle strength, especially of the quadriceps, is associated with severity of pain and low level of physical function [52, 54]. Psychological impairments such as pain catastrophizing [55], reduced pain coping skills [56], depression [57, 58], anxiety [57], and reduced social participation [58] are also associated with the severity of pain in individuals with knee OA. Furthermore, pain and physical and psychological impairments have shown bi-directional relationships, that is, physical and psychological impairments can influence, and in turn be influenced by severity of pain, results a further reduced physical and mental functioning [59].

5. Rehabilitation

Management of knee OA often requires a combination of pharmacologic and nonpharmacologic treatment approaches [60, 61]. Several clinical guidelines have been published by the scientific society for nonpharmacological treatment approach in knee OA [62–68]. Several randomized, controlled clinical trials have been published showing therapeutic effectiveness of exercise-based approaches, including range-of-motion exercises, aerobic exercise programs, and muscle-strengthening exercises [60, 61, 69, 70]. A previous study reported significant reduction in pain and functional disability scores of the Western Ontario and McMaster Universities (WOMAC) outcome measure following a home exercise program [69]. Another study reported significant reduction in pain following isometric quadriceps exercises for 3 months in knee OA [70]. Stitik et al. [71] had reported a significant reduction in pain intensity following combined use of hyaluronate injections and home exercise program in moderately severe pain in individuals with knee OA. Furthermore, previous randomized controlled studies reported that a simple quadriceps exercise performed at home was effective in reducing pain as well as functional disability [72, 73]. Another study reported a significant reduction in pain intensity and improved function following a simple group education program in patients with knee OA [74].

Passive treatment in the form of physiotherapeutic modalities such as short-wave diathermy, transcutaneous electrical nerve stimulation (TENS), ultrasound and hot packs often used to reduce both acute and chronic pain in knee OA [75]. However, Moffett et al. [76] reported that the short-wave diathermy had no additional benefits than placebo effects when used for 3 weeks in knee OA. In a recent published review, Zeng et al. [77] reported that the interferential current seems to be effective pain relief intervention in knee OA. Furthermore, they recommended that the other electrical stimulation therapy such as TENS, neuromuscular electrical stimulation, pulsed electrical stimulation, and noninvasive interactive neurostimulation is either uncertain or not appropriate for pain relief in knee OA [77].

Fransen and McConnell published a Cochrane review, in which, land-based therapeutic exercise (aerobic, resistance, stretching, strengthening, and range-of-motion exercises exercises) was compared with the non-exercise control group (home visits, education, waiting list, telephone call, relaxation, no intervention) in patients with hip or knee OA. The results of review indicate a significant reduction of self-reported pain and physical function for therapeutic exercise compared with control group [78]. Quadriceps strengthening is vital for alleviating pain and improving function in individuals with medial compartment knee OA [79]. Previous studies reported a reduced pain and improved function following knee flexors and extensors or hip abductors strengthening in knee OA [80–83]. Recently, a systematic review of 18 randomized controlled trials published, most of the included studies involved home-based exercise of quadriceps or lower extremity strengthening in knee OA. The results of this study indicate a significant reduction of pain and improvements in self-reported physical function following strengthening exercise in knee OA [79]. In another review, aerobic walking or home-based quadriceps-strengthening exercise was compared with a non-exercise control group in patients with knee OA. The results of review indicate both the types of exercise (aerobic walking or home-based quadriceps-strengthening exercise) significantly reduced knee pain compared with control group [84].

Cognitive behavioral therapy (CBT) is a psychological approach to train and enhance pain coping skills and found to be effective in reducing pain and improvement in self-efficacy in patients with knee OA [85–88]. CBT protocol includes three components: (i) patients education about the pain and the effect of pain coping skills on pain reduction, (ii) use of several cognitive and behavioral pain coping skills in a systematic manner, and (iii) the most challenging is to teach the patients how to use learned coping skills in a real-life situations [89]. A meta-analysis published recently had found that CBT is the most common studied psychosocial therapy approach for pain management in patients with arthritis [85]. Other studies recommended the use of pain coping skills training based on CBT, to reduce pain and improve psychological well-being in chronic pain conditions in patients with knee OA [90, 91].

Various other treatment techniques had shown significant effects on pain reduction in knee OA. Hinman et al. [92] reported significant reduction of pain following 3 weeks of therapeutic taping. Mulligan's mobilization with movement (MWM) technique seems to provide immediate pain relief and improved function in patients with knee OA [93]. Previous study recommended the use of laterally elevated wedge insoles inserting inside the shoes in patients with medial compartment knee OA [94]. Another study reported significant relief of pain using laterally elevated wedged insoles compared to neutrally wedged insoles in patients with knee OA [95]. However, other study reported no additional benefits of using braces and orthoses for the management of knee OA [96].

Acknowledgements

The Project was full financially supported by King Saud University, through Vice Deanship of Research Chairs, Rehabilitation Research Chair.

Author details

Shahnawaz Anwer[1,2*] and Ahmad Alghadir[1]

*Address all correspondence to: anwerphysio@gmail.com

1 Rehabilitation Research Chair, Department of Rehabilitation Sciences, College of Applied Medical Sciences, King Saud University, Riyadh, Saudi Arabia

2 Dr. D. Y. Patil College of Physiotherapy, Dr. D. Y. Patil Vidyapeeth, Pune, India

References

[1] Kim KW, Han JW, Cho HJ, Chang CB, Park JH, Lee JJ, Lee SB, Seong SC, Kim TK: Association between comorbid depression and osteoarthritis symptom severity in patients with knee osteoarthritis. J Bone Joint Surg Am. 2011;93(6):556–63. doi:10.2106/JBJS.I.01344

[2] Hinman RS, Hunt MA, Creaby MW, Wrigley TV, McManus FJ, Bennell KL: Hip muscle weakness in individuals with medial knee osteoarthritis. Arthritis Care Res (Hoboken). 2010;62(8):1190–3. doi:10.1002/acr.20199

[3] Heiden TL, Lloyd DG, Ackland TR: Knee extension and flexion weakness in people with knee osteoarthritis: is antagonist cocontraction a factor? J Orthop Sports Phys Ther. 2009;39(11):807–15. doi:10.2519/jospt.2009.3079

[4] Gupta S, Hawker GA, Laporte A, Croxford R, Coyte PC: The economic burden of disabling hip and knee osteoarthritis (OA) from the perspective of individuals living with this condition. Rheumatology (Oxford). 2005;44(12):1531–7. doi:10.1093/rheumatology/kei049

[5] Neogi T, Zhang Y: Epidemiology of osteoarthritis. Rheum Dis Clin N Am. 2013;39(1): 1–19. doi:10.1016/j.rdc.2012.10.004

[6] Childs JD, Sparto PJ, Fitzgerald GK, Bizzini M, Irrgang JJ: Alterations in lower extremity movement and muscle activation patterns in individuals with knee osteoarthritis. Clin Biomech (Bristol, Avon). 2004;19(1):44–9. doi:10.1016/j.clinbiomech.2003.08.007

[7] Liikavainio T, Lyytinen T, Tyrvainen E, Sipila S, Arokoski JP: Physical function and properties of quadriceps femoris muscle in men with knee osteoarthritis. Arch Phys Med Rehabil. 2008;89(11):2185–94. doi:10.1016/j.apmr.2008.04.012

[8] Liikavainio T, Bragge T, Hakkarainen M, Karjalainen PA, Arokoski JP: Gait and muscle activation changes in men with knee osteoarthritis. Knee. 2010;17(1):69–76. doi:10.1016/j.knee.2009.05.003

[9] Hinman RS, Bennell KL, Metcalf BR, Crossley KM: Delayed onset of quadriceps activity and altered knee joint kinematics during stair stepping in individuals with knee osteoarthritis. Arch Phys Med Rehabil. 2002;83(8):1080–6. doi:10.1053/apmr.2002.33068

[10] Loeser RF: Aging and osteoarthritis. Curr Opin Rheumatol. 2011;23(5):492–6. doi:10.1097/BOR.0b013e3283494005

[11] Silverwood V, Blagojevic-Bucknall M, Jinks C, Jordan JL, Protheroe J, Jordan KP. Current evidence on risk factors for knee osteoarthritis in older adults: a systematic review and meta-analysis. Osteoarthritis Cartilage. 2015;23(4):507–15. doi:10.1016/j.joca.2014.11.019

[12] Felson DT: Risk factors for osteoarthritis: understanding joint vulnerability. Clin Orthop Relat Res. 2004;427(Suppl):S16–21.

[13] Felson DT, Goggins J, Niu J, Zhang Y, Hunter DJ: The effect of body weight on progression of knee osteoarthritis is dependent on alignment. Arthritis Rheum. 2004;50(12):3904–9. doi:10.1002/art.20726

[14] O'Reilly SC, Jones A, Muir KR, Doherty M: Quadriceps weakness in knee osteoarthritis: the effect on pain and disability. Ann Rheum Dis. 1998;57(10):588–94. doi:10.1136/ard.57.10.588

[15] Slemenda C, Brandt KD, Heilman DK, Mazzuca S, Braunstein EM, Katz BP, Wolinsky FD: Quadriceps weakness and osteoarthritis of the knee. Ann Intern Med. 1997;127(2):97–104. Epub 1997/07/15. doi:10.7326/0003-4819-127-2-199707150-00001

[16] Kellgren JH, Lawrence JS: Radiological assessment of osteo-arthrosis. Ann Rheum Dis. 1957;16(4):494–502. doi:10.1136/ard.16.4.494

[17] Stevens-Lapsley JE, Kohrt WM: Osteoarthritis in women: effects of estrogen, obesity and physical activity. Womens Health (Lond Engl). 2010;6(4):601–15. doi:10.2217/whe.10.38

[18] Reid CR, Bush PM, Cummings NH, McMullin DL, Durrani SK: A review of occupational knee disorders. J Occup Rehabil. 2010;20(4):489–501. doi:10.1007/s10926-010-9242-8

[19] White DK, Zhang YQ, Felson DT, Niu JB, Keysor JJ, Nevitt MC, Lewis CE, Torner JC, Neogi T: The independent effect of pain in one versus two knees on the presence of low

physical function in a multicenter knee osteoarthritis study. Arthritis Care Res. 2010;62(7):938–43. doi:10.1002/acr.20166

[20] Fisher NM, Pendergast DR, Gresham GE, Calkins E: Muscle rehabilitation—its effect on muscular and functional performance of patients with knee osteoarthritis. Arch Phys Med Rehabil. 1991;72(6):365–74.

[21] Ettinger WH, Davis MA, Neuhaus JM, Mallon KP: Long-term physical functioning in persons with knee osteoarthritis from nhanes-I—effects of comorbid medical conditions. J Clin Epidemiol. 1994;47(7):809–15. doi:10.1016/0895-4356(94)90178-3

[22] Mcalindon TE, Cooper C, Kirwan JR, Dieppe PA: Determinants of disability in osteoarthritis of the knee. Ann Rheum Dis. 1993;52(4):258–62. doi:10.1136/ard.52.4.258

[23] Khaltaev N, Pfleger B, Woolf AD, Mathers C, Akesson K, Hazes JM, Symmons D: Assessing the burden of musculoskeletal conditions: a joint World Health Organization-Bone and Joint Decade project. Arthritis Res Ther. 2003;5(Suppl 3):174. doi:10.1186/ar805

[24] Blagojevic M, Jinks C, Jeffery A, Jordan KP: Risk factors for onset of osteoarthritis of the knee in older adults: a systematic review and meta-analysis. Osteoarthr Cartil. 2010;18(1):24–33. doi:10.1016/j.joca.2009.08.010

[25] Dawson J, Linsell L, Zondervan K, Rose P, Randall T, Carr A, Fitzpatrick R: Epidemiology of hip and knee pain and its impact on overall health status in older adults. Rheumatology (Oxford). 2004;43(4):497–504. doi:10.1093/rheumatology/keh086

[26] Felson DT, Hannan MT, Naimark A, Berkeley J, Gordon G, Wilson PW, Anderson J: Occupational physical demands, knee bending, and knee osteoarthritis—results from the Framingham-study. J Rheumatol. 1991;18(10):1587–92.

[27] Kujala UM, Kettunen J, Paananen H, Aalto T, Battie MC, Impivaara O, Videman T, Sarna S: Knee osteoarthritis in former runners, soccer players, weight lifters, and shooters. Arthritis Rheum. 1995;38(4):539–46. doi:10.1002/art.1780380413

[28] Wearing SC, Hennig EM, Byrne NM, Steele JR, Hills AP: Musculoskeletal disorders associated with obesity: a biomechanical perspective. Obes Rev. 2006;7(3):239–50. doi: 10.1111/j.1467-789X.2006.00251.x

[29] Brady TJ, Sniezek JE: Implementing the National Arthritis Action Plan: new population-based approaches to increasing physical activity among people with arthritis. Arthritis Rheum. 2003;49(3):471–6. doi:10.1002/art.11052

[30] Janke EA, Collins A, Kozak AT: Overview of the relationship between pain and obesity: what do we know? Where do we go next? J Rehabil Res Dev. 2007;44(2):245–62. doi: 10.1682/JRRD.2006.06.0060

[31] Anderson JJ, Felson DT: Factors associated with osteoarthritis of the knee in the first national Health and Nutrition Examination Survey (HANES I). Evidence for an

association with overweight, race, and physical demands of work. Am J Epidemiol. 1988;128(1):179–89.

[32] Leach RE, Baumgard S, Broom J: Obesity: its relationship to osteoarthritis of the knee. Clin Orthop Relat Res. 1973;93:271–3.

[33] Hartz AJ, Fischer ME, Bril G, Kelber S, Rupley D, Jr., Oken B, Rimm AA: The association of obesity with joint pain and osteoarthritis in the HANES data. J Chronic Dis. 1986;39(4):311–9. doi:10.1016/0021-9681(86)90053-6

[34] Griffin TM, Guilak F: The role of mechanical loading in the onset and progression of osteoarthritis. Exerc Sport Sci Rev. 2005;33(4):195–200. doi:0091-6331/3304/195–200

[35] Zhai G, Blizzard L, Srikanth V, Ding C, Cooley H, Cicuttini F, Jones G: Correlates of knee pain in older adults: Tasmanian Older Adult Cohort Study. Arthritis Rheum. 2006;55(2):264–71. doi:10.1002/art.21835

[36] Slemenda C, Heilman DK, Brandt KD, Katz BP, Mazzuca SA, Braunstein EM, Byrd D: Reduced quadriceps strength relative to body weight: a risk factor for knee osteoarthritis in women? Arthritis Rheum. 1998;41(11):1951–9. doi: 10.1002/1529-0131(199811)41:11<1951

[37] Segal NA, Torner JC, Felson D, Niu J, Sharma L, Lewis CE, Nevitt M: Effect of thigh strength on incident radiographic and symptomatic knee osteoarthritis in a longitudinal cohort. Arthritis Rheum. 2009;61(9):1210–7. doi:10.1002/art.24541

[38] Palmieri-Smith RM, Thomas AC, Karvonen-Gutierrez C, Sowers MF: Isometric quadriceps strength in women with mild, moderate, and severe knee osteoarthritis. Am J Phys Med Rehabil. 2010;89(7):541–8. doi:10.1097/PHM.0b013e3181ddd5c3

[39] Segal NA, Glass NA: Is quadriceps muscle weakness a risk factor for incident or progressive knee osteoarthritis? Phys Sportsmed. 2011;39(4):44–50. doi:10.3810/psm. 2011.11.1938

[40] Hunter DJ, Felson DT: Osteoarthritis. BMJ. 2006;332(7542):639–42. doi:10.1136/bmj. 332.7542.639

[41] Kijowski R, Blankenbaker D, Stanton P, Fine J, De Smet A: Arthroscopic validation of radiographic grading scales of osteoarthritis of the tibiofemoral joint. AJR Am J Roentgenol. 2006;187(3):794–9. doi:10.2214/AJR.05.1123

[42] Altman R, Asch E, Bloch D, Bole G, Borenstein D, Brandt K, Christy W, Cooke TD, Greenwald R, Hochberg M, et al.: Development of criteria for the classification and reporting of osteoarthritis. Classification of osteoarthritis of the knee. Diagnostic and Therapeutic Criteria Committee of the American Rheumatism Association. Arthritis Rheum. 1986;29(8):1039–49. doi:10.1002/art.1780290816

[43] Dieppe PA, Lohmander LS: Pathogenesis and management of pain in osteoarthritis. Lancet. 2005;365(9463):965–73. doi:10.1016/S0140-6736(05)71086-2

[44] Davis MA, Ettinger WH, Neuhaus JM, Mallon KP: Knee osteoarthritis and physical functioning: evidence from the NHANES I Epidemiologic Followup Study. J Rheumatol. 1991;18(4):591–8.

[45] Sayre EC, Li LC, Kopec JA, Esdaile JM, Bar S, Cibere J: The effect of disease site (knee, hip, hand, foot, lower back or neck) on employment reduction due to osteoarthritis. Plos one. 2010;5(5):e10470. doi:10.1371/journal.pone.0010470

[46] Kaufman KR, Hughes C, Morrey BF, Morrey M, An KN: Gait characteristics of patients with knee osteoarthritis. J Biomech. 2001;34(7):907–15. doi:10.1016/S0021-9290(01)00036-7

[47] Hurley MV, Scott DL, Rees J, Newham DJ: Sensorimotor changes and functional performance in patients with knee osteoarthritis. Ann Rheum Dis. 1997;56(11):641–8. doi:10.1136/ard.56.11.641

[48] McCloskey DI: Kinesthetic sensibility. Physiol Rev. 1978;58(4):763–820.

[49] Carvalho NA, Bittar ST, Pinto FR, Ferreira M, Sitta RR: Manual for guided home exercises for osteoarthritis of the knee. Clinics (Sao Paulo). 2010;65(8):775–80.doi: 10.1590/S1807-59322010000800006

[50] Easton BT: Evaluation and treatment of the patient with osteoarthritis. J Fam Pract. 2001;50(9):791–7.

[51] Creamer P, Hochberg MC: The relationship between psychosocial variables and pain reporting in osteoarthritis of the knee. Arthritis Care Res. 1998;11(1):60–5.

[52] Sharma L, Cahue S, Song J, Hayes K, Pai YC, Dunlop D: Physical functioning over three years in knee osteoarthritis: role of psychosocial, local mechanical, and neuromuscular factors. Arthritis Rheum. 2003;48(12):3359–70. doi:10.1002/art.11420

[53] Dieppe PA: Relationship between symptoms and structural change in osteoarthritis: what are the important targets for therapy? J Rheumatol. 2005;32(6):1147–9.

[54] Eitzen I, Holm I, Risberg MA: Preoperative quadriceps strength is a significant predictor of knee function two years after anterior cruciate ligament reconstruction. Br J Sports Med. 2009;43(5):371–6. doi:10.1136/bjsm.2008.057059

[55] Somers TJ, Keefe FJ, Pells JJ, Dixon KE, Waters SJ, Riordan PA, Blumenthal JA, McKee DC, LaCaille L, Tucker JM, Schmitt D, Caldwell DS, Kraus VB, Sims EL, Shelby RA, Rice JR: Pain catastrophizing and pain-related fear in osteoarthritis patients: relationships to pain and disability. J Pain Symptom Manag. 2009;37(5):863–72. doi:10.1016/j.jpainsymman.2008.05.009

[56] van Baar ME, Dekker J, Lemmens JA, Oostendorp RA, Bijlsma JW: Pain and disability in patients with osteoarthritis of hip or knee: the relationship with articular, kinesiological, and psychological characteristics. J Rheumatol. 1998;25(1):125–33.

[57] Smith BW, Zautra AJ: The effects of anxiety and depression on weekly pain in women with arthritis. Pain. 2008;138(2):354–61. doi:10.1016/j.pain.2008.01.008

[58] Rosemann T, Laux G, Szecsenyi J, Wensing M, Grol R: Pain and osteoarthritis in primary care: factors associated with pain perception in a sample of 1,021 patients. Pain Med. 2008;9(7):903–10. doi:10.1111/j.1526-4637.2008.00498.x

[59] Sale JE, Gignac M, Hawker G: The relationship between disease symptoms, life events, coping and treatment, and depression among older adults with osteoarthritis. J Rheumatol. 2008;35(2):335–42.

[60] Recommendations for the medical management of osteoarthritis of the hip and knee—2000 update. American College of Rheumatology Subcommittee on Osteoarthritis Guidelines. Arthritis Rheum. 2000;43(9):1905–15.

[61] Pendleton A, Arden N, Dougados M, Doherty M, Bannwarth B, Bijlsma JWJ, Cluzeau F, Cooper C, Dieppe PA, Günther KP, et al.: EULAR recommendations for the management of knee osteoarthritis: report of a task force of the Standing Committee for International Clinical Studies Including Therapeutic Trials (ESCISIT). Ann Rheum Dis. 2000;59(12):936–44. doi:10.1136/ard.59.12.936

[62] Hochberg MC, Altman RD, Brandt KD, Clark BM, Dieppe PA, Griffin MR, Moskowitz RW, Schnitzer TJ: Guidelines for the medical management of osteoarthritis. Part I. Osteoarthritis of the hip. American College of Rheumatology. Arthritis Rheum. 1995;38(11):1535–40. doi:10.1002/art.1780381103

[63] Hochberg MC, Altman RD, Brandt KD, Clark BM, Dieppe PA, Griffin MR, Moskowitz RW, Schnitzer TJ: Guidelines for the medical management of osteoarthritis. Part II. Osteoarthritis of the knee. American College of Rheumatology. Arthritis Rheum. 1995;38(11):1541–6. doi:10.1002/art.1780381104

[64] Roddy E, Zhang W, Doherty M, Arden NK, Barlow J, Birrell F, Carr A, Chakravarty K, Dickson J, Hay E, et al.: Evidence-based recommendations for the role of exercise in the management of osteoarthritis of the hip or knee—the MOVE consensus. Rheumatology (Oxford). 2005;44(1):67–73. doi:10.1093/rheumatology/keh399

[65] Mazieres B, Bannwarth B, Dougados M, Lequesne M: EULAR recommendations for the management of knee osteoarthritis. Report of a task force of the Standing Committee for International Clinical Studies Including Therapeutic Trials. Joint Bone Spine. 2001;68(3):231–40. doi:10.1016/S1297-319X(01)00271-8

[66] Ottawa panel evidence-based clinical practice guidelines for therapeutic exercises and manual therapy in the management of osteoarthritis. Phys Ther. 2005;85(9):907–71. http://ptjournal.apta.org/content/85/9/907

[67] Hunter DJ: Quality of osteoarthritis care for community-dwelling older adults. Clin Geriatr Med. 2010;26(3):401–17. doi:10.1016/j.cger.2010.03.003

[68] Brand CA, Ackerman IN, Bohensky MA, Bennell KL: Chronic disease management: a review of current performance across quality of care domains and opportunities for

improving osteoarthritis care. Rheum Dis Clin N Am. 2013;39(1):123–43. doi:10.1016/j.rdc.2012.10.005

[69] Thomas KS, Muir KR, Doherty M, Jones AC, O'Reilly SC, Bassey EJ: Home based exercise programme for knee pain and knee osteoarthritis: randomised controlled trial. BMJ. 2002;325(7367):752–5. doi:10.1136/bmj.325.7367.752

[70] Miyaguchi M, Kobayashi A, Kadoya Y, Ohashi H, Yamano Y, Takaoka K: Biochemical change in joint fluid after isometric quadriceps exercise for patients with osteoarthritis of the knee. Osteoarthr Cartil. 2003;11(4):252–9. doi:10.1016/S1063-4584(02)00372-2

[71] Stitik TP, Blacksin MF, Stiskal DM, Kim JH, Foye PM, Schoenherr L, Choi ES, Chen B, Saunders HJ, Nadler SF: Efficacy and safety of hyaluronan treatment in combination therapy with home exercise for knee osteoarthritis pain. Arch Phys Med Rehabil. 2007;88(2):135–41. doi:10.1016/j.apmr.2006.11.006

[72] Petrella RJ, Bartha C: Home based exercise therapy for older patients with knee osteoarthritis: a randomized clinical trial. J Rheumatol. 2000;27(9):2215–21.

[73] O'Reilly SC, Muir KR, Doherty M: Effectiveness of home exercise on pain and disability from osteoarthritis of the knee: a randomised controlled trial. Ann Rheum Dis. 1999;58(1):15–9. doi:10.1136/ard.58.1.15

[74] Bezalel T, Carmeli E, Katz-Leurer M: The effect of a group education programme on pain and function through knowledge acquisition and home-based exercise among patients with knee osteoarthritis: a parallel randomised single-blind clinical trial. Physiotherapy. 2010;96(2):137–43. doi:10.1016/j.physio.2009.09.009.

[75] Cetin N, Aytar A, Atalay A, Akman MN: Comparing hot pack, short-wave diathermy, ultrasound, and TENS on isokinetic strength, pain, and functional status of women with osteoarthritic knees: a single-blind, randomized, controlled trial. Am J Phys Med Rehabil. 2008;87(6):443–51. doi:10.1097/PHM.0b013e318174e467

[76] Moffett JA, Richardson PH, Frost H, Osborn A: A placebo controlled double blind trial to evaluate the effectiveness of pulsed short wave therapy for osteoarthritic hip and knee pain. Pain. 1996;67(1):121–7. doi:10.1016/0304-3959(96)03100-4

[77] Zeng C, Li H, Yang T, Deng ZH, Yang Y, Zhang Y, Lei GH. Electrical stimulation for pain relief in knee osteoarthritis: systematic review and network meta-analysis. Osteoarthr Cartil. 2015;23(2):189–202. doi:10.1016/j.joca.2014.11.014

[78] Fransen M, McConnell S: Exercise for osteoarthritis of the knee. Cochrane Database Syst Rev. 2008;4:CD004376. doi:10.1002/14651858.CD004376.pub2

[79] Lange AK, Vanwanseele B, Singh MA: Strength training for treatment of osteoarthritis of the knee: a systematic review. Arthritis Rheum. 2008;59(10):1488–94. doi:10.1002/art.24118

[80] Bennell KL, Hunt MA, Wrigley TV, Hunter DJ, McManus FJ, Hodges PW, Li L, Hinman RS: Hip strengthening reduces symptoms but not knee load in people with medial knee

osteoarthritis and varus malalignment: a randomised controlled trial. Osteoarthr Cartil. 2010;18(5):621–8. doi:10.1016/j.joca.2010.01.010

[81] Lim BW, Kemp G, Metcalf B, Wrigley TV, Bennell KL, Crossley KM, Hinman RS: The association of quadriceps strength with the knee adduction moment in medial knee osteoarthritis. Arthritis Rheum. 2009;61(4):451–8. doi:10.1002/art.24278

[82] King LK, Birmingham TB, Kean CO, Jones IC, Bryant DM, Giffin JR: Resistance training for medial compartment knee osteoarthritis and malalignment. Med Sci Sports Exerc. 2008;40(8):1376–84. doi:10.1249/MSS.0b013e31816f1c4a

[83] Sled EA, Khoja L, Deluzio KJ, Olney SJ, Culham EG: Effect of a Home program of hip abductor exercises on knee joint loading, strength, function, and pain in people with knee osteoarthritis: a clinical trial. Phys Ther. 2010;90(6):895–904. doi:10.2522/ptj.20090294

[84] Roddy E, Zhang W, Doherty M: Aerobic walking or strengthening exercise for osteoarthritis of the knee? A systematic review. Ann Rheum Dis. 2005;64(4):544–8. doi:10.1136/ard.2004.028746

[85] Dixon KE, Keefe FJ, Scipio CD, Perri LM, Abernethy AP: Psychological interventions for arthritis pain management in adults: a meta-analysis. Health Psychol. 2007;26(3): 241–50. doi:10.1037/0278-6133.26.3.241

[86] Keefe FJ, Blumenthal J, Baucom D, Affleck G, Waugh R, Caldwell DS, Beaupre P, Kashikar-Zuck S, Wright K, Egert J, Lefebvre J: Effects of spouse-assisted coping skills training and exercise training in patients with osteoarthritic knee pain: a randomized controlled study. Pain. 2004;110(3):539–49. doi:10.1016/j.pain.2004.03.022

[87] Keefe FJ, Caldwell DS, Baucom D, Salley A, Robinson E, Timmons K, Beaupre P, Weisberg J, Helms M: Spouse-assisted coping skills training in the management of knee pain in osteoarthritis: long-term followup results. Arthritis Care Res. 1999;12(2):101–11.

[88] Keefe FJ, Caldwell DS, Williams DA, Gil KM, Mitchell D, Robertson C, et al. Pain coping skills training in the management of osteoarthritic knee pain —a comparative-study. Behav Ther. 1990;21(1):49–62.

[89] Hunt MA, Keefe FJ, Bryant C, Metcalf BR, Ahamed Y, Nicholas MK, Bennell KL: A physiotherapist-delivered, combined exercise and pain coping skills training intervention for individuals with knee osteoarthritis: a pilot study. Knee. 2013;20(2):106–12. doi:10.1016/j.knee.2012.07.008

[90] Devos-Comby L, Cronan T, Roesch SC: Do exercise and self-management interventions benefit patients with osteoarthritis of the knee? A metaanalytic review. J Rheumatol. 2006;33(4):744–56.

[91] Hurley MV, Walsh NE: Effectiveness and clinical applicability of integrated rehabilitation programs for knee osteoarthritis. Curr Opin Rheumatol. 2009;21(2):171–6. doi: 10.1097/BOR.0b013e3283244422

[92] Hinman RS, Crossley KM, McConnell J, Bennell KL: Efficacy of knee tape in the management of osteoarthritis of the knee: blinded randomised controlled trial. BMJ. 2003;327(7407):135. doi:10.1136/bmj.327.7407.135

[93] Takasaki H, Hall T, Jull G: Immediate and short-term effects of Mulligan's mobilization with movement on knee pain and disability associated with knee osteoarthritis—a prospective case series. Physiother Theory Pract. 2013;29(2):87–95. doi: 10.3109/09593985.2012.702854

[94] Reilly KA, Barker KL, Shamley D: A systematic review of lateral wedge orthotics—how useful are they in the management of medial compartment osteoarthritis? Knee. 2006;13(3):177–83. doi:10.1016/j.knee.2006.02.003

[95] Hatef MR, Mirfeizi Z, Sahebari M, Jokar MH, Mirheydari M: Superiority of laterally elevated wedged insoles to neutrally wedged insoles in medial knee osteoarthritis symptom relief. Int J Rheum Dis. 2014;17(1):84–8. doi:10.1111/1756-185X.12036

[96] Brouwer RW, Jakma TS, Verhagen AP, Verhaar JA, Bierma-Zeinstra SM: Braces and orthoses for treating osteoarthritis of the knee. Cochrane Database Syst Rev. 2005;1:CD004020. doi:10.1002/14651858.CD004020.pub2

Chapter 6

Application of Radiofrequency in Pain Management

Suleyman Deniz, Omer Bakal and Gokhan Inangil

Additional information is available at the end of the chapter

http://dx.doi.org/10.5772/100803

Abstract

The application of radiofrequency is a treatment for many clinical conditions such as trigeminal neuralgia, complex regional pain syndrome, chronic postsurgical pain, cancer pain, hyperhidrosis and facet joint pain requiring ablation of different nerve locations. In this procedure, a constant high-frequency, high-temperature electrical current is applied to target tissue. Sluijter has achieved significant pain relief using radiofrequency current at a temperature below 42°C that produced strong electromagnetic field with no thermal lesion and referred as pulsed radiofrequency. The use of pulsed radiofrequency is a non-neurodestructive and therefore less painful technique, and it serves as an alternative method to continuous radiofrequency. Many studies have demonstrated favorable outcomes with pulsed radiofrequency compared to continuous radiofrequency.

This chapter suggests the use of continuous and pulsed radiofrequency with a minimally invasive procedure for patients with chronic pain as an alternative to surgical treatment and it might be an additional option among nonsurgical treatment methods.

Keywords: pain, treatment, pulsed radiofrequency, minimally invasive surgical procedures, continuous

1. Introduction

The application of radiofrequency (RF) electrical signals to neural tissue with an RF lesion generator and RF electrodes inserted into the tissue is common to treat pain [1] and other diseases such as atrial fibrillation [2], malignant liver tumors [3], intermediate and large bone tumors [4] and varicose veins [5]. The basis of this method is to generate enough RF heating power in the tissue to raise the temperature above 45–50°C which is referred as the "lethal temperature", as the tissue exposed to these temperatures for 20 s or more are known to be destroyed by the heat [1].

The earliest RF lesion generators and electrodes were built by Cosman et al. in the early 1950s. They used continuous-wave RF with 0.1–1 mHz frequency and therefore referred as continuous RF lesioning [6, 7]. The basic principles and properties such as shape and size of heat lesions caused by for different electrode geometries and temperatures are well described today [8].

Recently, another RF method is especially used for pain treatment in which short pulses of RF signals are applied to the neural tissue through the RF electrode. This method is referred as pulsed RF lesioning [9].

While continuous RF used power sources with 0.1–1 mHz frequency range to produce RF heat lesion, pulsed RF signals have pulse durations ranging from 10 to 30 ms, and pulse repetition rates ranging from 1 to 8 Hz (pulses per second) [1]. Pulsed RF which produces a lesion to nerve tissue by transmission of high-voltage current through thermocouple probe has been used as a non- or minimally neurodestructive technique alternative to heat lesions because the average tissue temperature rise is less than continuous RF with the same voltage [1, 10–14]. Sluijter has achieved significant pain relief using radiofrequency current at a temperature below 42°C that produced strong electromagnetic field with no thermal lesion [9–11].

The objective of this book chapter is to explain the physics, operating principles, the mechanism of action, contraindications, complications and evaluation of efficacy of pulsed RF and continuous RF therapies in chronic pain management, in addition discussion of examples of clinical procedures.

2. The physics and operating principles of radiofrequency

RF lesioning is based on the principle of a very-high-frequency current passage down a 27G thermocouple probe which is inserted through a special 22G fully insulated cannula except for its tip. The current passes down the thermocouple probe and heats the surrounding tissues to a temperature controlled by the operator. The location of the nerve is achieved by a stimulating current with the thermocouple probe, and with a destructive current a circumscribed lesion is created. The lesion is shaped like a match with a diameter of about 2–4 mm [1, 11, 12].

The cannula, placed close to the targeted nerve to be lesioned, is usually confirmed under X-ray. Then, stylet of cannula is removed and replaced by the thermocouple probe. The operator initially attempts to seek the nerve by low-voltage stimulation at a frequency of 50 Hz, aiming the strongest sensory stimulation at the lowest possible voltage. The cannula needs to be within 3 mm of the nerve in order to create an adequate lesion and a maximum stimulation level of around 0.6 V would indicate this. The operator should always ensure that the cannula is not dangerously close to any motor nerve when trying to lesion a sensory nerve [1, 10–12].

When the operator is satisfied that the needle is in a safe place, a radiofrequency current (about 300–500 kHz) is passed through the thermocouple probe. The current heats up the surrounding tissues and produces a lesion in the targeted nerve. At a temperature of below 44–50°C, no permanent neurological damage will occur; thus, for practical purposes, when we mention lesion size, we mean the volume of tissue within the 44–50°C. In all cell types, the heating of tissue above 44–50°C for several minutes will indeed result in cell death [1, 10–12].

In order to eliminate any possibility of a heat lesion being produced, Sluijter suggested a radiofrequency technique which uses a temperature of no greater than 42°C and which utilises the strong electric field generated by the passage of the radiofrequency current to achieve pain relief [12]. In order to apply an electric field to the tissues, without raising the tip temperature above 42°C, the radiofrequency current can be applied in a pulsed fashion. The "silent" period between pulses allows for the dissipation of heat produced during the active cycle [12]. Cosman and Sluijter have modified the standard lesion generator to deliver radiofrequency current bursts of 45 V at a repetition rate of 2 Hz with each burst 20 ms long; the rest period is therefore 480 msec. This is defined as pulsed RF [10–12, 15, 16].

The resistance to the current flow can be measured and it is useful in certain procedures since it indicates the position of the needle tip. The impedans will be 400 Ω in extradural tissues and measuring a 200 will warn operator that the tip is passed to the cerebrospinal fluid (CSF) and a 800 Ω impedans will indicate when the tip enters CSF during percutaneuous cordotomy. Similarly, during procedures with intervertebral disc, an impedans is very high and it falls below 200 Ω while nucleus pulposus impedans of nucleus pulposus is reached [1, 10–12].

3. Mechanism of action of radiofrequency

Continuous RF lesioning involves the passage of a very high frequency which causes destruction by heat. It is simple and clear. Efficacy of pulsed RF has been clinically documented and has been used for chronic pain conditions for the last 20 years, but its mechanism of action is not fully understood [10–14]. It has been suggested to alter gene expression in neurons, by means of neuromodulation [1, 11, 17–23]. Stimulation of serotonergic and noradrenergic systems and induction of descending pathways have also been proposed [22]. There is no clinical evidence of any nerve damage with pulsed RF [11, 12, 19, 22, 23]. Higuchi et al. have presented experimental evidence that pulsed RF applied to the rat cervical dorsal root ganglion causes upregulation of the immediate early gene c-fos immunoreactivity in the laminae I & II of the dorsal horn [18]. Hamann et al. applied pulsed RF to the sciatic nerve or the L5 dorsal root ganglion in the rat. They studied the expression of activating transmission factor 3 (ATF3), an early intermediate gene expressed in response to cell stress. They also reported a trend downregulation of CGRP expression [24]. Hamann et al., pointing out the lack of laboratory evidence for this phenomenon, felt that this may be due to changes induced in the function of the Schwann cells [24]. Electric fields have demonstrated effects on immune modulation, as there are studies that show proinflammatory cytokines, such as interleukin (IL)-1b, TNF-alpha and IL-6, are attenuated by electric fields [25]. Upregulation of adenosine A2A receptor density has also been observed in human neutrophils treated with generated electric fields, and this appeared to be associated with inhibition of the catabolic cytokines, such as TNF-alpha, IL-6 and IL-8 [26].

In an animal study evaluating the histologic effects of continuous RF at 67°C and pulsed RF applied adjacent to rabbit dorsal root ganglia (DRG), Erdine et al. found mitochondrial degeneration and a loss of nuclear membrane integrity in the continuous, but not in the pulsed group [27]. Another histopathologic study, comparing the effects of continuous RF and pulsed RF delivered at 42°C on the rat DRG and sciatic nerve, showed no structural changes aside from transient endoneurial edema and collagen deposition [28]. In addition, Hagiwara et al. more recently demonstrated that pulsed RF may actually enhance the descending noradrenergic and serotonergic inhibitory pathways, which are intimately involved in the modulation of neuropathic pain [22]. Pulsed RF may be useful and continuous RF is contraindicated, e.g., in neuropathic pain and it is safe in locations where continuous RF may be potentially hazardous, e.g., DRG lesioning. It is virtually painless as no heat is generated [10–12].

Sluijter describes four phases in a pulsed RF treatment procedure:

a. *A stunning phase, which provides immediate relief.*

b. *A phase of post procedure discomfort, which may last for up to 3 weeks.*

c. *A phase of beneficial clinical effect, which has a variable duration.*

d. *A phase of recurrence of pain, we are still in the early days but many cases record 4–24 months of relief* [11, 12].

4. Contraindications of radiofrequency

Gauci does not recommend the use of both continuous and pulsed RF in patients with psychological overlay, drug dependency and total body pain [12]. Continuous RF treatment is also contraindicated in all nerve that carries motor fibers [1, 10–13].

Pulsed RF therapy seems ineffective in some diseases and would be contraindicated. Whereas according to some studies, pulsed RF appears to be ineffective in our opinion; one of the reasons for this is the insufficient "pulsed RF dose" applied. For example, in a study the anti-allodynic effects of pulsed RF was significantly greater when pulsed RF exposure was increased from 2 to 6 min [29]. Therefore, there also exist unresolved questions regarding the effective "pulsed RF dose" based on voltage settings and duration of pulsed RF treatment, which require further clinical studies in order to confirm.

5. Complications of radiofrequency

The high temperature applied with continuous RF is neurodestructive and is usually characterized by a period of discomfort, including hypoanesthesia and a neuritis-like reaction [1, 10–14]. Sometimes pain may potentially worsen due to nerve regeneration and may lead to neuroma formation. Other complications such as hematoma, numbness, transitory diplopia, meningitis, Horner's syndrome and urinary retention may occur [12–14, 16, 17, 19, 30, 31].

In the publication of Cahana et al., it is stated that there is documentation of more than 1200 patients who have been treated with pulsed RF and no neurological complication was reported [23]. In a recent clinical study on patients with premature ejaculation, pulsed RF was performed to dorsal nerves of penis and no functional disorder that indicates a nerve lesion was determined [19]. We have not observed such a complication in our clinical experience.

6. Procedure for application of radiofrequency

The applications of continuous and pulsed RF in our department were made in operating room. Before procedure, prothrombin time and platelet counts were checked. Following a peripheral IV route, the patients were monitorized with ECG, oxygen saturation and non-invasive arterial blood pressure and sedated with 0.02 mg/kg IV midazolam. Following subcutaneous local anesthetic infiltration, a RF lesion generator was used for continuous and pulsed RF thermal ablation. A 22-gauge, 5–15 cm, RF cannula with a 2–10 mm active-pinned tip (with matching electrode) is advanced to the target tissue. The electrode of the RF device is placed on the cannula, and the impedance is seen to be between 200–400 Ω. In order to check the position of the cannula neurophysiologically, paresthesia is observed with 50 Hz sensory stimulation at 0.3–0.5 V and lack of motor contraction with 2 Hz motor stimulation at 0.9–1.5 V. After this neurophysiological testing, continuous RF thermal coagulation is applied at 60–80°C for 60–120 s. Pulsed RF thermal coagulation is applied at 42°C for 120–600 s. Following thermal coagulation, 2 ml of 2% lidocaine is applied through the cannula. All patients are monitored for potential complications following 2 h after the procedure. Patients were discharged home on the same day.

7. Applications of radiofrequency treatment

a. Radiofrequency facet joint denervation

- *Cervical facet joint denervation* [12, 32–35]

  Target: Medial branch of the cervical posterior primary ramus

  Required equipment: Mobile C-arm fluoroscopic X-ray systems, RF lesion generator, the cannula (a 22-gauge, 5 cm length, 2–4 mm active-curved tip (with matching electrode) of the RF, the grounding line

  Patient position: Supine and the X-ray tube "looks" at the side opposite to that being treated (C2–C5), prone (C6–C7)

  View: Lateral-oblique view of the cervical spine (C2–C5), postero-anterior-oblique view of the cervical spine (C6–C7)

Treatment modality: Continuous RF (80°C for 60 s), pulsed RF (42°C for 120–360 s)

- *Thoracic facet joint denervation* [12, 32, 34, 35]

  Target: Medial branch of the thoracic posterior primary ramus

  Required equipment: Mobile C-arm fluoroscopic X-ray systems, RF lesion generator, the cannula (a 22-gauge, 5–10 cm length, 2–4 mm active-curved tip (with matching electrode) of the RF, the grounding line

  Patient position: Prone

  View: Postero-anterior view of the thoracic spine

  Treatment modality: Continuous RF (80–85°C for 60 s), pulsed RF (42°C for 120–360 s)

- *Lumbar facet joint denervation* [12, 32, 34–36]

  Target: Medial branch of the lumbar posterior primary ramus (eye of the Scottie dog, L1–L4), the junction between the superior articular process and the upper surface of the lateral part of the sacrum (L5), just lateral to the sacral foramen (S1–S3)

  Required equipment: Mobile C-arm fluoroscopic X-ray systems, RF lesion generator, the cannula (a 22-gauge, 10–15 cm length, 5 mm active-pinned tip (with matching electrode) of the RF, the grounding line

  Patient position: Prone

  View: Postero-anterior-oblique view of the lumbar spine (tunnel vision)

  Treatment modality: Continuous RF (85°C for 60 s), pulsed RF (42°C for 180–360 s)

b. Radiofrequency dorsal root ganglion

- *Cervical DRG pulsed RF/continuous RF* [12, 34, 35, 37]

  Target: Typical cervical DRG (C3–C6)

  Required equipment: Mobile C-arm fluoroscopic X-ray systems, RF lesion generator, the cannula (a 22-gauge, 5–10 cm length, 2 mm active-curved tip (with matching electrode) of the RF, the grounding line

  Patient position: Supine and the X-ray tube "looks" at the side opposite to that being treated (C1–C6), prone (C7–C8)

  View: Lateral-oblique view of the cervical spine (C2–C5), postero-anterior-oblique view of the cervical spine (C6–C7)

  Treatment modality: Pulsed RF (42°C for 120 s), continuous RF (65°C for 60 s) (do not carry out C1–C2)

  Attention: The vertebral artery may lie in needle path. Careful! (C1–C2)

http://dx.doi.org/10.5772/100803

- *Thoracic DRG pulsed RF/continuous RF* [12, 34, 38–40]

  Information: Effective in the treatment of chronic thoracic postherpetic neuralgia and chronic postsurgical thoracic pain

  Target: Thoracic DRG

  Required equipment: Mobile C-arm fluoroscopic X-ray systems, RF lesion generator, the cannula (a 22-gauge, 10 cm length, 2 mm active-curved tip (with matching electrode) of the RF, the grounding line

  Patient position: Prone

  View: Postero-anterior-oblique view of the thoracic spine, angle your beam slightly cranially (T1–6), angle your beam slightly caudally (T7–12)

  Treatment modality: Pulsed RF (42°C for 120 s), continuous RF (67°C for 60 s)

  Attention: Pneumothorax! Careful!

- *Lumbar DRG pulsed RF/continuous RF* [12, 27, 41–43]

  Information: Effective in the treatment of chronic post-amputation stump pain and complex regional pain syndrome

  Target: Lumbar DRG

  Required equipment: Mobile C-arm fluoroscopic X-ray systems, RF lesion generator, the cannula (a 22-gauge, 10–15 cm length, 2 mm active-pinned tip (with matching electrode) of the RF, the grounding line

  Patient position: Prone

  View: Postero-anterior-oblique view of the lumbar spine (no double end plate) (chin of the dog)

  Treatment modality: Pulsed RF (42°C for 120 s), continuous RF (50–65°C for 60 s)

c. Radiofrequency sympathetic nervous system

- *Sphenopalatine ganglion pulsed RF/continuous RF* [12, 44–47]

  Information: Effective in the treatment of posttraumatic headache, chronic face and head pain and cluster headaches

  Target: Pterygopalatine fossa, pterygomaxillary fissure

  Required equipment: Mobile C-arm fluoroscopic X-ray systems, RF lesion generator, the cannula (a 22-gauge, 5 cm length, 2 mm active-pinned tip (with matching electrode) of the RF, the grounding line

  Patient position: Supine and the X-ray tube "looks" at opposite to the treated side

  View: Lateral-oblique X-ray view of skull to show pterygomaxillary fissure

Treatment modality: Pulsed RF (42°C for 120–240 s), continuous RF (60–90°C for 60–90 s)

- *Superior cervical ganglion pulsed RF/continuous RF* [12, 48]

  Information: Effective in the treatment of tinnitus and atypical face pain

  Target: The superior cervical sympathetic ganglion is formed by the coalescence of the upper four cervical sympathetic ganglia. It is situated at the level of C3, postero-medial to the carotid sheath and to the internal jugular vein

  Required equipment: Mobile C-arm fluoroscopic X-ray systems, RF lesion generator, the cannula (a 22-gauge, 5–10 cm length, 2 mm active-curved tip (with matching electrode) of the RF, the grounding line

  Patient position: Prone

  View: Lateral-oblique X-ray view of the cervical spine

  Treatment modality: Pulsed RF (42°C for 120 s), continuous RF (70–75°C for 60 s)

- *Stellate ganglion pulsed RF/continuous RF* [12, 49–51]

  Information: Effective in the treatment of complex regional pain syndrome and posttraumatic stress disorder

  Target: It is situated at the level of C7

  Required equipment: Mobile C-arm fluoroscopic X-ray systems, RF lesion generator, the cannula (a 22-gauge, 5–10 cm length, 2 mm active-curved tip (with matching electrode) of the RF, the grounding line

  Patient position: Supine, prevent patient swallowing during procedure!

  View: Antero-posterior X-ray view of the cervical spine

  Treatment modality: Pulsed RF (42°C for 120 s), continuous RF (70–75°C for 60 s)

  Attention: Ask the patient to phonate (recurrent laryngeal nerve!), Horner's syndrome!

- *Thoracic sympathetic ganglion pulsed RF/continuous RF* [12, 52–54]

  Information: Effective in the treatment of complex regional pain syndrome, palmar hyperhidrosis and compensatory hyperhidrosis of the trunk

  Target: It is situated at the levels of T4, T2, T3 and T6

  Required equipment: Mobile C-arm fluoroscopic X-ray systems, RF lesion generator, the cannula (a 22-gauge, 5–10 cm length, 2 mm active-curved tip (with matching electrode) of the RF, the grounding line

  Patient position: Prone

  View: Postero-anterior X-ray view of the thoracic spine

Treatment modality: Pulsed RF (42°C for 120 s), continuous RF (75–80°C for 60–90 s)

Attention: Pneumothorax!

- *Splanchnic nerve pulsed RF/continuous RF* [12, 55–58]

  Information: Effective in the treatment of chronic abdominal pain, chronic pancreatitis and cancer pain

  Target: It is situated at the level of T11 at the costovertebral angle (about 4 cm from the midline)

  Required equipment: Mobile C-arm fluoroscopic X-ray systems, RF lesion generator, the cannula (a 22-gauge, 15 cm length, 2–5 mm active-curved tip (with matching electrode) of the RF, the grounding line

  Patient position: Prone

  View: Postero-anterior X-ray view of the thoracic spine

  Treatment modality: Pulsed RF (42°C for 120 s), continuous RF (75–80°C for 60–90 s)

  Attention: Pneumothorax!

- *Lumbar sympathetic ganglion continuous RF/pulsed RF* [12, 59–61]

  Information: Effective in the treatment of complex regional pain syndrome, plantar hyperhidrosis, chronic pelvic and perineal pain and cancer pain

  Target: It is situated at the level of L4, L2 and L3

  Required equipment: Mobile C-arm fluoroscopic X-ray systems, RF lesion generator, the cannula (a 22-gauge, 15 cm length, 2–5 mm active-pinned tip (with matching electrode) of the RF, the grounding line

  Patient position: Prone

  View: Postero-anterior-oblique and lateral X-ray view of the lumbar spine (no double end plate)

  Treatment modality: Continuous RF (80°C for 90 s), pulsed RF (42°C for 120–300 s)

d. Miscellaneous procedures

- *Trigeminal ganglion continuous RF/pulsed RF* [12, 62–64]

  Information: Effective in the trigeminal neuralgia treatment of combined pulsed and continuous radiofrequency

  Target: Foramen ovale

  Required equipment: Mobile C-arm fluoroscopic X-ray systems, RF lesion generator, the cannula (a 22-gauge, 10 cm length, 2–5 mm active-pinned tip (with matching electrode) of the RF, the grounding line

Patient position: Supine

View: X-ray beam in an antero-posterior axis over the head, move the axis of the intensifier caudo-cranially so that the X-ray beam makes an angle of 45°, next, 45–50° between the sagittal and the vertical planes. Lateral control (Clivus must be seen!)

Treatment modality: Continuous RF (60°C for 60 s, followed by; 65°C for 60 s, followed by; 70°C for 60 s, followed by; 75°C for 60 s, and next, 80°C for 60 s), pulsed RF (42°C for 120–240 s)

Attention: The procedure is very painful (Sedoanalgesia may be required!), CSF may be seen (If so, position is correct). Exhibit eye movements or facial contractions may be seen (If so, position is incorrect), blood may be seen (If so, position is incorrect), contractions of the masseter muscles can be seen (If so, position is incorrect), corneal reflex should be protected!

- *Intradiscal RF/pulsed RF* [12, 65, 66]

  Target: Posterior anulus tear

  Required equipment: Mobile C-arm fluoroscopic X-ray systems, RF lesion generator, the cannula (a 22-gauge, 15 cm length, 2–5 mm active-pinned tip (with matching electrode) of the RF, the grounding line

  Patient position: Prone

  View: Postero-anterior-oblique view of the lumbar spine (no double end plate)

  Treatment modality: Continuous RF (50°C for 120 s, followed by; 55°C for 120 s, followed by; 60°C for 120 s, and next; 65°C for 240 s), pulsed RF (42°C for 120–900 s)

  Attention: Monitor external temperature of disc, never exceeds 44°C

- *Occipital nerve pulsed RF* [12, 67, 68]

  Information: Effective in the treatment of occipital neuralgia, migraine and cervicogenic headaches

  Target: Greater occipital nerve (C2), lesser occipital nerve (C3)

  Required equipment: RF lesion generator, the cannula (a 22-gauge, 5 cm length, 4 mm active-pinned tip (with matching electrode) of the RF, the grounding line, ultrasonography

  Patient position: The sitting position

  View: Occipital artery can be viewed with ultrasonography

  Treatment modality: Pulsed RF (42°C for 180–600 s)

  Attention: Temperature not to exceed 42°C

- *Suprascapular nerve pulsed RF* [12, 69–71]

  Information: Effective in the treatment of adhesive capsulitis, chronic shoulder pain

  Target: Suprascapular notch

  Required equipment: RF lesion generator, the cannula (a 22-gauge, 10 cm length, 5 mm active-pinned tip (with matching electrode) of the RF, the grounding line, ultrasonography

  Patient position: The sitting position

  View: Suprascapular artery can be viewed with ultrasonography

  Treatment modality: Pulsed RF (42°C for 180–600 s)

  Attention: Temperature not to exceed 42°C, Be careful about pneumothorax!

- *Percutaneous cervical cordotomy* [12, 72–74]

  Information: Indicated for unilateral pain due to malignant disease, when the pain is not responsive to drug therapy or other less invasive methods of treatment. The patient cannot be sedated

  Target: C1/C2 intervertebral space, lateral spinothalamic tract

  Required equipment: RF lesion generator, the cannula (a 22-gauge, 5–10 cm length, 2 mm active-pinned tip (with matching electrode) of the RF (Cordotomy kit!), the grounding line, computerized tomography

  Patient position: Supine

  View: Lateral view of cervical spine

  Treatment modality: Continuous RF (75°C for 60 s, followed by; 75°C for 60 s, followed by; 75°C for 60 s, and next; 75°C for 60 s)

  Attention: Working on the side opposite to the pain! Protect motor fibers!

Also, pulsed RF are reported in the literature that it can be used in treatment of *Morton's neuroma* [13], *coccygodynia* [14], *pudendal neuralgia* [75], *vaginismus* [76], *carpal tunnel syndrome* [77], *chronic hip pain* [78], *post herniorrhaphy pain* [79], *chronic inguinal neuralgia* [80], *plantar heel pain* [81], *osteoarthritis* [82], *intra-articular pain* [83], *plantar fascitis pain* [84], *tarsal tunnel syndrome* [85], *myofascial pain syndrome* [86], *postamputation phantom pain* [87], *meralgia paresthetica* [88], *lingual neuralgia* [89] and *chronic testicular pain* [90].

This chapter suggests the use of continuous and pulsed RF with a minimally invasive procedure for patients with chronic pain as an alternative to surgical treatment and it might be an additional option among non-surgical treatment methods. On the other hand, further randomized prospective controlled studies in patients with chronic pain are needed to fully evaluate the effectiveness of continuous and pulsed RF.

Author details

Suleyman Deniz*, Omer Bakal and Gokhan Inangil

*Address all correspondence to: sdeniz.md@gmail.com

Gulhane Military Medical Academy, Haydarpasa Training Hospital, Department of Anesthesiology, Pain Management Unit, Istanbul, Turkey

References

[1] Cosman ER Jr, Cosman ER Sr. Electric and thermal field effects in tissue around radiofrequency electrodes. Pain Med. 2005;6:405–24.

[2] Hunter RJ, Baker V, Finlay MC, Duncan ER, Lovell MJ, Tayebjee MH, Ullah W, Siddiqui MS, McLEAN A, Richmond L, Kirkby C, Ginks MR, Dhinoja M, Sporton S, Earley MJ, Schilling RJ. Point-by-point radiofrequency ablation versus the cryoballoon or a novel combined approach: a randomized trial comparing 3 methods of pulmonary vein isolation for paroxysmal atrial fibrillation (the cryo versus RF trial). J Cardiovasc Electrophysiol. 2015;26:1307–14. doi: 10.1111/jce.12846.

[3] Lencioni R, de Baere T, Martin RC, Nutting CW, Narayanan G. Image-guided ablation of malignant liver tumors: recommendations for clinical validation of novel thermal and non-thermal technologies - a western perspective. Liver Cancer. 2015;4:208–14. doi: 10.1159/000367747.

[4] Nakatsuka A, Yamakado K, Uraki J, Takaki H, Yamanaka T, Fujimori M, Hasegawa T, Sakuma H. Safety and clinical outcomes of percutaneous radiofrequency ablation for intermediate and large bone tumors using a multiple-electrode switching system: a phase ii clinical study. J Vasc Interv Radiol. 2015 Dec 23. pii: S1051-0443(15)01068-4. doi: 10.1016/j.jvir.2015.10.025.

[5] Kim J, Cho S, Joh JH, Ahn HJ, Park HC. Effect of diameter of saphenous vein on stump length after radiofrequency ablation for varicose vein. Vasc Specialist Int. 2015;31:125–9. doi: 10.5758/vsi.2015.31.4.125.

[6] Cosman BJ, Cosman ER. Guide to Radio Frequency Lesion Generation in Neurosurgery. Burlington, MA: Radionics; 1974.

[7] Cosman ER, Cosman BJ. Methods of making nervous system lesions. In: Wilkens RH, Rengachary SS, eds. Neurosurgery. New York: McGraw-Hill; 1984:2490–9.

[8] Cosman ER, Nashold BS, Ovelman-Levitt J. Theoretical aspects of radiofrequency lesions in the dorsal root entry zone. Neurosurgery. 1984;15:945–50.

[9] Sluijter ME, Cosman ER, Rittman WJ, Van Kleef M. The effects of pulsed radiofrequency fields applied to the dorsal root ganglion: a preliminary report. The Pain Clinic. 1998;II(2):109–17.

[10] Chua NH, Vissers KC, Sluijter ME. Pulsed radiofrequency treatment in interventional pain management: mechanisms and potential indications-a review. Acta Neurochir (Wien). 2011;153:763–71. doi: 10.1007/s00701-010-0881-5.

[11] Sluijter ME. Pulsed radiofrequency. In Radiofrequency, Part 1. Fliovopress SA, Meggen (LU), Switzerland; 2001. 55–68.

[12] Gauci CA. The Manual of RF-Techniques. Flivo Press SA, Meggen (LU), Switzerland; 2004. 8–140.

[13] Deniz S, Purtuloglu T, Tekindur S, Cansız KH, Yetim M, Kılıckaya O, Senkal S, Bilgic S, Atim A, Kurt E. Ultrasound-guided pulsed radio frequency treatment in Morton's neuroma. J Am Podiatr Med Assoc. 2015;105:302–6. doi: 10.7547/13-128.1.

[14] Atim A, Ergin A, Bilgiç S, Deniz S, Kurt E. Pulsed radiofrequency in the treatment of coccygodynia. Agri. 2011;23:1–6.

[15] Cosman ER. A comment on the history of the pulsed radiofrequency technique for pain therapy. Anesthesiology. 2005;103:1312.

[16] Sluijter ME, van Kleef M. Pulsed radiofrequency. Pain Med. 2007;8:388–9; author reply 390–1.

[17] van Boxem K, van Eerd M, Brinkhuizen T, Patijn J, van Kleef M, van Zundert J. Radiofrequency and pulsed radiofrequency treatment of chronic pain syndromes: the available evidence. Pain Pract. 2008;8:385–93.

[18] Higuchi Y, Nashold BS Jr, Sluijter M, Cosman E, Pearlstein RD. Exposure of the dorsal root ganglion in rats to pulsed radiofrequency currents activates dorsal horn lamina I and II neurons. Neurosurgery 2002;50:850–5; discussion 856.

[19] Basal S, Goktas S, Ergin A, Yildirim I, Atim A, Tahmaz L, Dayanc M. A novel treatment modality in patients with premature ejaculation resistant to conventional methods: the neuromodulation of dorsal penile nerves by pulsed radiofrequency. J Androl. 2010;31:126–30.

[20] Munglani R. The longer term effect of pulsed radiofrequency for neuropathic pain. Pain. 1999;80:437–9.

[21] Richebé P, Rathmell JP, Brennan TJ. Immediate early genes after pulsed radiofrequency treatment: neurobiology in need of clinical trials. Anesthesiology. 2005;102:1–3.

[22] Hagiwara S, Iwasaka H, Takeshima N, Noguchi T. Mechanisms of analgesic action of pulsed radiofrequency on adjuvant induced pain in the rat: roles of descending adrenergic and serotonergic systems. Eur J Pain. 2009;13:249–52.

[23] Cahana A, Van Zundert J, Macrea L, van Kleef M, Sluijter M. Pulsed radiofrequency: current clinical and biological literature available. Pain Med. 2006;7:411–23.

[24] Hamann W, Abou-Sherif S, Thompson S, Hall S. Pulsed radiofrequency applied to dorsal root ganglia causes a selective increase in ATF3 in small neurons. Eur J Pain. 2006;10:171–6.

[25] Igarashi A, Kikuchi S, Konno S. Correlation between inflammatory cytokines released from the lumbar facet joint tissue and symptoms in degenerative lumbar spinal disorders. J Orthop Sci. 2007;12:154–60.

[26] Varani K, Gessi S, Merighi S, Iannotta V, Cattabriga E, Spisani S, Cadossi R, Borea PA. Effect of low frequency electromagnetic fields on A2A adenosine receptors in human neutrophils. Br J Pharmacol. 2002;136:57–66.

[27] Erdine S, Yucel A, Cimen A, Aydin S, Sav A, Bilir A. Effects of pulsed versus conventional radiofrequency current on rabbit dorsal root ganglion morphology. Eur J Pain. 2005;9:251–6.

[28] Podhajsky RJ, Sekiguchi Y, Kikuchi S, Myers RR. The histologic effects of pulsed and continuous radiofrequency lesions at 42 degrees C to rat dorsal root ganglion and sciatic nerve. Spine (Phila Pa 1976). 2005;30:1008–13.

[29] Tanaka N, Yamaga M, Tateyama S, Uno T, Tsuneyoshi I, Takasaki M. The effect of pulsed radiofrequency current on mechanical allodynia induced with resiniferatoxin in rats. Anesth Analg. 2010;111:784–90. doi: 10.1213/ANE.0b013e3181e9f62f.

[30] Rozen D, Parvez U. Pulsed radiofrequency of lumbar nerve roots for treatment of chronic inguinal herniorraphy pain. Pain Physician. 2006;9:153–6.

[31] Bogduk N. Pulsed radiofrequency. Pain Med. 2006;7:396–407.

[32] Manchikanti L, Kaye AD, Boswell MV, Bakshi S, Gharibo CG, Grami V, Grider JS, Gupta S, Jha SS, Mann DP, Nampiaparampil DE, Sharma ML, Shroyer LN, Singh V, Soin A, Vallejo R, Wargo BW, Hirsch JA. A systematic review and best evidence synthesis of the effectiveness of therapeutic facet joint interventions in managing chronic spinal pain. Pain Physician. 2015;18:E535–82.

[33] Liliang PC, Lu K, Hsieh CH, Kao CY, Wang KW, Chen HJ. Pulsed radiofrequency of cervical medial branches for treatment of whiplash-related cervical zygapophysial joint pain. Surg Neurol. 2008;70(Suppl 1):S1:50–5; discussion S1:55. doi: 10.1016/j.surneu.2008.07.006.

[34] van Kleef M, Stolker RJ, Lataster A, Geurts J, Benzon HT, Mekhail N. Thoracic pain. Pain Pract. 2010;10:327–38. doi: 10.1111/j.1533-2500.2010.00376.x.

[35] Manchikanti L, Abdi S, Atluri S, Benyamin RM, Boswell MV, Buenaventura RM, Bryce DA, Burks PA, Caraway DL, Calodney AK, Cash KA, Christo PJ, Cohen SP, Colson J, Conn A, Cordner H, Coubarous S, Datta S, Deer TR, Diwan S, Falco FJ, Fellows B, Geffert S, Grider JS, Gupta S, Hameed H, Hameed M, Hansen H, Helm S 2nd, Janata

JW, Justiz R, Kaye AD, Lee M, Manchikanti KN, McManus CD, Onyewu O, Parr AT, Patel VB, Racz GB, Sehgal N, Sharma ML, Simopoulos TT, Singh V, Smith HS, Snook LT, Swicegood JR, Vallejo R, Ward SP, Wargo BW, Zhu J, Hirsch JA. An update of comprehensive evidence-based guidelines for interventional techniques in chronic spinal pain. Part II: guidance and recommendations. Pain Physician. 2013;16(2 Suppl):S49–283.

[36] Koh W, Choi SS, Karm MH, Suh JH, Leem JG, Lee JD, Kim YK, Shin J. Treatment of chronic lumbosacral radicular pain using adjuvant pulsed radiofrequency: a randomized controlled study. Pain Med. 2015;16:432–41. doi: 10.1111/pme.12624.

[37] Yoon YM, Han SR, Lee SJ, Choi CY, Sohn MJ, Lee CH. The efficacy of pulsed radiofrequency treatment of cervical radicular pain patients. Korean J Spine. 2014;11:109–12. doi: 10.14245/kjs.2014.11.3.109.

[38] Ke M, Yinghui F, Yi J, Xeuhua H, Xiaoming L, Zhijun C, Chao H, Yingwei W. Efficacy of pulsed radiofrequency in the treatment of thoracic postherpetic neuralgia from the angulus costae: a randomized, double-blinded, controlled trial. Pain Physician. 2013;16:15–25.

[39] van Kleef M, Barendse GA, Dingemans WA, Wingen C, Lousberg R, de Lange S, Sluijter ME. Effects of producing a radiofrequency lesion adjacent to the dorsal root ganglion in patients with thoracic segmental pain. Clin J Pain. 1995;11:325–32.

[40] Cohen SP, Sireci A, Wu CL, Larkin TM, Williams KA, Hurley RW. Pulsed radiofrequency of the dorsal root ganglia is superior to pharmacotherapy or pulsed radiofrequency of the intercostal nerves in the treatment of chronic postsurgical thoracic pain. Pain Physician. 2006;9:227–35.

[41] Nagda JV, Davis CW, Bajwa ZH, Simopoulos TT. Retrospective review of the efficacy and safety of repeated pulsed and continuous radiofrequency lesioning of the dorsal root ganglion/segmental nerve for lumbar radicular pain. Pain Physician. 2011;14:371–6.

[42] Ramanavarapu V, Simopoulos TT. Pulsed radiofrequency of lumbar dorsal root ganglia for chronic post-amputation stump pain. Pain Physician. 2008;11:561–6.

[43] Apiliogullari S, Aydin BK, Onal O, Kirac Y, Celik JB. Pulsed radiofrequency of dorsal root ganglia for the treatment of complex regional pain syndrome in an adolescent with poliomyelitis sequel: a case report. Pain Med. 2015;16:1369–72. doi: 10.1111/pme.12710.

[44] Shah RV, Racz GB. Long-term relief of posttraumatic headache by sphenopalatine ganglion pulsed radiofrequency lesioning: a case report. Arch Phys Med Rehabil. 2004;85:1013–6.

[45] Day M. Neurolysis of the trigeminal and sphenopalatine ganglions. Pain Pract. 2001;1:171–82.

[46] Bayer E, Racz GB, Miles D, Heavner J. Sphenopalatine ganglion pulsed radiofrequency treatment in 30 patients suffering from chronic face and head pain. Pain Pract. 2005;5:223–7.

[47] Fang L, Jingjing L, Ying S, Lan M, Tao W, Nan J. Computerized tomography-guided sphenopalatine ganglion pulsed radiofrequency treatment in 16 patients with refractory cluster headaches: twelve- to 30-month follow-up evaluations. Cephalalgia. 2015 Apr 20. pii: 0333102415580113.

[48] Koning HM, Dyrbye BA, van Hemert FJ. Percutaneous radiofrequency lesion of the superior cervical sympathetic ganglion in patients with tinnitus. Pain Pract. 2015 Aug 27. doi: 10.1111/papr.12348.

[49] Martin DC, Willis ML, Mullinax LA, Clarke NL, Homburger JA, Berger IH. Pulsed radiofrequency application in the treatment of chronic pain. Pain Pract. 2007;7:31–5.

[50] Lipov E. Successful use of stellate ganglion block and pulsed radiofrequency in the treatment of posttraumatic stress disorder: a case report. Pain Res Treat. 2010;2010:963948. doi: 10.1155/2010/963948.

[51] van Eijs F, Stanton-Hicks M, Van Zundert J, Faber CG, Lubenow TR, Mekhail N, van Kleef M, Huygen F. Evidence-based interventional pain medicine according to clinical diagnoses. 16. Complex regional pain syndrome. Pain Pract. 2011;11:70–87. doi: 10.1111/j.1533-2500.2010.00388.x.

[52] Purtuloğlu T, Deniz S, Atım A, Tekindur Ş, Gürkök S, Kurt E. A new target of percutaneous sympathetic radiofrequency thermocoagulation for treatment of palmar hyperhidrosis: T4. Agri. 2013;25:36–40. doi: 10.5505/agri.2013.09226.

[53] Purtuloglu T, Atim A, Deniz S, Kavakli K, Sapmaz E, Gurkok S, Kurt E, Turan A. Effect of radiofrequency ablation and comparison with surgical sympathectomy in palmar hyperhidrosis. Eur J Cardiothorac Surg. 2013;43:e151–4. doi: 10.1093/ejcts/ezt024.

[54] Deniz S, Kavaklı K, Çaylak H, Purtuloğlu T, Sapmaz E, İnangil G, Atım A, Gürkök S, Kurt E. Treatment of compensatory hyperhidrosis of the trunk with radiofrequency ablation. Agri. 2015;27:42–6. doi: 10.5505/agri.2015.37167.

[55] Raj PP, Thomas J, Heavner J, Racz G, Lou L, Day M, Shaw BC. The development of a technique for radiofrequency lesioning of splanchnic nerves. Curr Rev Pain. 1999;3:377–387.

[56] Garcea G, Thomasset S, Berry DP, Tordoff S. Percutaneous splanchnic nerve radiofrequency ablation for chronic abdominal pain. ANZ J Surg. 2005;75:640–4.

[57] Gangi A, Buy X, Garnon J, Tsoumakidou G, Moser T, Bierry G, Muller A. Pain management in oncology. J Radiol. 2011;92:801–13. doi: 10.1016/j.jradio.2011.07.014.

[58] Verhaegh BP, van Kleef M, Geurts JW, Puylaert M, van Zundert J, Kessels AG, Masclee AA, Keulemans YC. Percutaneous radiofrequency ablation of the splanchnic nerves in

patients with chronic pancreatitis: results of single and repeated procedures in 11 patients. Pain Pract. 2013;13:621–6. doi: 10.1111/papr.12030.

[59] Aşik ZS, Orbey BC, Aşik I. Sympathetic radiofrequency neurolysis for unilateral lumbar hyperhidrosis: a case report. Agri. 2008;20:37–9.

[60] Straube S, Derry S, Moore RA, McQuay HJ. Cervico-thoracic or lumbar sympathectomy for neuropathic pain and complex regional pain syndrome. Cochrane Database Syst Rev. 2010 Jul 7;(7):CD002918. doi: 10.1002/14651858.CD002918.pub2.

[61] Rigaud J, Delavierre D, Sibert L, Labat JJ. Sympathetic nerve block in the management of chronic pelvic and perineal pain. Prog Urol. 2010;20:1124–31. doi: 10.1016/j.purol.2010.08.047.

[62] Zhao WX, Wang Q, He MW, Yang LQ, Wu BS, Ni JX. Radiofrequency thermocoagulation combined with pulsed radiofrequency helps relieve postoperative complications of trigeminal neuralgia. Genet Mol Res. 201513;14:7616–23. doi: 10.4238/2015.July.13.5.

[63] Ali Eissa AA, Reyad RM, Saleh EG, El-Saman A. The efficacy and safety of combined pulsed and conventional radiofrequency treatment of refractory cases of idiopathic trigeminal neuralgia: a retrospective study. J Anesth. 2015;29:728–33. doi: 10.1007/s00540-015-2029-5.

[64] Thapa D, Ahuja V, Dass C, Verma P. Management of refractory trigeminal neuralgia using extended duration pulsed radiofrequency application. Pain Physician. 2015;18:E433–5.

[65] Fukui S, Nitta K, Iwashita N, Tomie H, Nosaka S, Rohof O. Intradiscal pulsed radiofrequency for chronic lumbar discogenic low back pain: a one year prospective outcome study using discoblock for diagnosis. Pain Physician. 2013;16:E435–42.

[66] Kapural L, Vrooman B, Sarwar S, Krizanac-Bengez L, Rauck R, Gilmore C, North J, Girgis G, Mekhail N. A randomized, placebo-controlled trial of transdiscal radiofrequency, biacuplasty for treatment of discogenic lower back pain. Pain Med. 2013;14:362–73. doi: 10.1111/pme.12023.

[67] Hamer JF, Purath TA. Response of cervicogenic headaches and occipital neuralgia to radiofrequency ablation of the C2 dorsal root ganglion and/or third occipital nerve. Headache. 2014;54:500–10. doi: 10.1111/head.12295.

[68] Cohen SP, Peterlin BL, Fulton L, Neely ET, Kurihara C, Gupta A, Mali J, Fu DC, Jacobs MB, Plunkett AR, Verdun AJ, Stojanovic MP, Hanling S, Constantinescu O, White RL, McLean BC, Pasquina PF, Zhao Z. Randomized, double-blind, comparative-effectiveness study comparing pulsed radiofrequency to steroid injections for occipital neuralgia or migraine with occipital nerve tenderness. Pain. 2015;156:2585–94. doi: 10.1097/j.pain.0000000000000373.

[69] Keskinbora K, Aydinli I. Long-term results of suprascapular pulsed radiofrequency in chronic shoulder pain. Agri. 2009;21:16–21.

[70] Gofeld M, Restrepo-Garces CE, Theodore BR, Faclier G. Pulsed radiofrequency of suprascapular nerve for chronic shoulder pain: a randomized double-blind active placebo-controlled study. Pain Pract. 2013;13:96–103. doi: 10.1111/j.1533-2500.2012.00560.x.

[71] Wu YT, Ho CW, Chen YL, Li TY, Lee KC, Chen LC. Ultrasound-guided pulsed radiofrequency stimulation of the suprascapular nerve for adhesive capsulitis: a prospective, randomized, controlled trial. Anesth Analg. 2014;119:686–92. doi: 10.1213/ANE.0000000000000354.

[72] Lippe PM. Neurosurgery-epitomes of progress: percutaneous radiofrequency cervical cordotomy: treatment of chronic intractable pain. West J Med. 1977;127:233–4.

[73] Raslan AM. Percutaneous computed tomography-guided radiofrequency ablation of upper spinal cord pain pathways for cancer-related pain. Neurosurgery. 2008;62(3 Suppl 1):226–33; discussion 233–4. doi: 10.1227/01.neu.0000317397.16089.f5.

[74] Fonoff ET, Lopez WO, de Oliveira YS, Teixeira MJ. Microendoscopy-guided percutaneous cordotomy for intractable pain: case series of 24 patients. J Neurosurg. 2015 Jul 31:1–8.

[75] Hong MJ, Kim YD, Park JK, Hong HJ. Management of pudendal neuralgia using ultrasound-guided pulsed radiofrequency: a report of two cases and discussion of pudendal nerve block techniques. J Anesth. 2015 Dec 23.

[76] Carvalho JC, Agualusa LM, Moreira LM, Costa JC. Multimodal therapeutic approach of vaginismus: an innovative approach through trigger point infiltration and pulsed radiofrequency of the pudendal nerve. Rev Bras Anestesiol. 2015 Nov 30. pii: S0034–7094(15)00047-1. doi: 10.1016/j.bjan.2014.10.005.

[77] Chen LC, Ho CW, Sun CH, Lee JT, Li TY, Shih FM, Wu YT. Ultrasound-guided pulsed radiofrequency for carpal tunnel syndrome: a single-blinded randomized controlled study. PLoS One. 2015;10:e0129918. doi: 10.1371/journal.pone.0129918. eCollection 2015.

[78] Chye CL, Liang CL, Lu K, Chen YW, Liliang PC. Pulsed radiofrequency treatment of articular branches of femoral and obturator nerves for chronic hip pain. Clin Interv Aging. 2015;10:569–74. doi: 10.2147/CIA.S79961. eCollection 2015.

[79] Gupta M, Gupta P. Ultrasound out of plane approach for pulsed radiofrequency treatment of post herniorrhaphy pain: synchronizing treatment and imaging modality. Saudi J Anaesth. 2015;9:224–5. doi: 10.4103/1658-354X.152897.

[80] Makharita MY, Amr YM. Pulsed radiofrequency for chronic inguinal neuralgia. Pain Physician. 2015;18:E147-55.

[81] Ye L, Mei Q, Li M, Gu M, Ai Z, Tang K, Shi D, Wu X, Wang X, Zheng Y. A comparative efficacy evaluation of ultrasound-guided pulsed radiofrequency treatment in the

gastrocnemius in managing plantar heel pain: a randomized and controlled trial. Pain Med. 2015;16:782–90. doi: 10.1111/pme.12664.

[82] Rahimzadeh P, Imani F, Faiz SH, Entezary SR, Nasiri AA, Ziaeefard M. Investigation the efficacy of intra-articular prolotherapy with erythropoietin and dextrose and intra-articular pulsed radiofrequency on pain level reduction and range of motion improvement in primary osteoarthritis of knee. J Res Med Sci. 2014;19:696–702.

[83] Eyigor C, Eyigor S, Akdeniz S, Uyar M. Effects of intra-articular application of pulsed radiofrequency on pain, functioning and quality of life in patients with advanced knee osteoarthritis. J Back Musculoskelet Rehabil. 2015;28:129–34.

[84] Thapa D, Ahuja V. Combination of diagnostic medial calcaneal nerve block followed by pulsed radiofrequency for plantar fascitis pain: a new modality. Indian J Anaesth. 2014;58:183–5. doi: 10.4103/0019-5049.130824.

[85] Chon JY, Hahn YJ, Sung CH, Jung SH, Moon HS. Pulsed radiofrequency under ultrasound guidance for the tarsal tunnel syndrome: two case reports. J Anesth. 2014;28:924–7. doi: 10.1007/s00540-014-1831-9.

[86] Niraj G. Ultrasound-guided pulsed radiofrequency treatment of myofascial pain syndrome: a case series. Br J Anaesth. 2012;109:645–6. doi: 10.1093/bja/aes331.

[87] Imani F, Gharaei H, Rezvani M. Pulsed radiofrequency of lumbar dorsal root ganglion for chronic postamputation phantom pain. Anesth Pain Med. 2012;1:194–7. doi: 10.5812/kowsar.22287523.3768.

[88] Choi HJ, Choi SK, Kim TS, Lim YJ. Pulsed radiofrequency neuromodulation treatment on the lateral femoral cutaneous nerve for the treatment of meralgia paresthetica. J Korean Neurosurg Soc. 2011;50:151–3. doi: 10.3340/jkns.2011.50.2.151.

[89] Rehman SU, Khan MZ, Hussain R, Jamshed A. Pulsed radiofrequency modulation for lingual neuralgia. Br J Oral Maxillofac Surg. 2012;50:e4–5. doi: 10.1016/j.bjoms.2011.06.001.

[90] Misra S, Ward S, Coker C. Pulsed radiofrequency for chronic testicular pain-a preliminary report. Pain Med. 2009;10:673–8. doi: 10.1111/j.1526-4637.2009.00581.x.

Chapter 7

Epiduroscopy (Epidural Endoscopy)

Havva Sayhan and Serbulent Gokhan Beyaz

Additional information is available at the end of the chapter

http://dx.doi.org/10.5772/62918

Abstract

Epiduroscopy is a relatively new technique used in the evaluation and treatment of low back pain via advancements in optical fiber technology. As a minimally invasive endoscopic technique, it allows for direct endoscopic imaging of the epidural space and helps the patients for the pain management who having post–lumbar surgery syndrome (PLSS) and other cases of low back pain and radiculopathy. An advanced understanding of the anatomy of epidural space and adjacent structures are also essential for positive and successful clinical outcomes. The use of epiduroscopy in the pain clinic is performed as a day procedure, and the patient is awake and can communicate with the doctor. During an epiduroscopy, thin tubes with a bright light and tiny fiberoptic camera at the end are inserted through the sacral hiatus into the epidural space around the dura and guided up toward the affected site. Anterior epiduroscopy and epiduroscopic laser neural decompression (ELND) have been recently introduced in treating herniated disc decompressions, and chronic low back pain and radicular pain, respectively. The most common complications of epiduroscopic approach are the pain in the intervention point, dural puncture, and headache.

Keywords: epiduroscopy, anterior epiduroscopy, epiduroscopic laser discectomy, post–lumbar surgery syndrome (PLSS), low back pain, chronic pain, epidural space

1. Introduction

Epiduroscopy, also known as spinal endoscopy, which is directly visualize the epidural space with a percutaneously minimal invasive inserted fiberoptic scope. Epiduroscopy is a relatively new diagnostic and therapeutic technique developed in the [1] performed to treat the low back pain, specifically radicular pain in which the epidural space is directly visualized on a video monitor. The development of epiduroscopy is connected to the integration of fiber-optic technology with computer-enhanced imaging for viewing the central nervous system that is miniaturized enough to be inserted into the epidural space. The fiber-optic visualization would be easy and safe to apply in medical practice and has made a major contribution to advances in pain medicine. In this way, the epidural space can be identified for the cause of pain and other neurological signs by distinguishing the anatomic structures and pathological structures.

Epiduroscopy involves looking inside the epidural space that contains nerves who are pain generators inside of the spinal column that connect the spinal cord to the rest of the body. An epiduroscopy involves insertion of a tiny fiber-optic camera attached to a catheter into the epidural space through a small incision in the sacral hiatus near the tail bone. The areas of concern can then be visualized by guided up towards the affected nerve roots. Afterward, the adhesions can be cut away and local anesthetic and steroid solutions can be injected.

The increased attention has been paid to epiduroscopy to deliver accurate diagnosis and treatment for chronic pain. Recently, as a result of these efforts, epiduroscopically assisted laser therapy has been reported for multiple lesions such as discectomy [2]. Epiduroscopy is expected to provide successful outcomes in the diagnosis and treatment of intractable low back and leg pain where even epidural steroid injection is not efficacious for pain relief and pain recurs after operation.

2. History of epiduroscopy

Epiduroscopy was considered a method to study the spinal anatomy, and then improvements allowed its employment as therapeutic approach in the diagnosis and treatment of pain. Clinicians have been working with various types of endoscopes for over 80 years, with varying degrees of success.

In the 1930s, Burman started the first study on epiduroscopy and reported direct visualization of the spinal canal with arthroscopic equipment to examine the anatomy of the vertebral column that were removed intact from human cadavers [3].

The first use of the instrument on patients did by Stern in1936 for the direct observation of the posterior roots for rhizotomies and for the treatment of spastic conditions.

Later, Pool developed this system which did not have any recording and imaging system and applied the technique clinically on over 400 patients. He could diagnose conditions such as neuritis, herniated disc, neoplasms, adhesions, and venous congestion [4].

Afterward, researchers focused on visualizing the spinal canal, however, there was no further remarkable progress on endoscopy in the literature until the late 1950s.

The key breakthrough for clinical application of this technology is the development of the first flexible endoscope in 1958 by Hirschowitz et al. [5] that gave rise to enormous advances in diagnostics and therapy.

In the late 1960s and early 1970s, the Japanese researcher Ooi and Morisaki [6] developed an instrument for intradural and extradural examinations that combined a flexible light source with rigid optics. The fiber-optic light source technology protected the tissues from heat injury, since the fibers absorb infrared rays and reflect visible rays.

In 1991, Saberski and Kitahata [7] considered clinical use of these devices for the placement into the epidural space as a diagnostic tool where the caudal approach to the epidural space offer advantage over the paramedian lumbar approach. The authors reported that the caudal approach facilitated correct catheter positioning for administration of epidural steroid for the treatment of radiculopathy.

In 1993, Leu et al. [8] used endoscopies for therapeutic intervention in addition to diagnostics, and performed peridural and intraductal endoscopies in patients.

Schutze et al. [9] conducted the first video-optic examinations of the lumbar epidural space in chronic patients with a flexible catheter-secured epiduroscopic unit.

Epiduroscopy received approval through the United States Food and Drug Administration (FDA) in 1996 for visualization of the epidural space.

Recently, minimal invasive and microsurgical techniques such as epiduroscopic laser discectomy have been introduced and used for chronic low back pain and post–lumbar surgery syndrome (PLSS) which was called before as false back surgery syndrome (FBSS). Considering the ongoing development trends in the area of microsystems technology, epidural endoscopy has an increasing significance of invasive intervention in pain medicine.

3. Indications and contraindications

The pain physician's major responsibilities involve treating unexplained pain symptoms and effective pain management. It can be difficult to classify and treat chronic spinal pain syndromes.

Therefore, the conformity between clinical examination, imaging results, diagnostic blocks, and epiduroscopy is the backbone to ascertain the cause of pain and to establish a diagnosis in clinical decision.

Epiduroscopy has the advantage of visually identified structures in the epidural space such as hyperemia, changes in vascularity, fibrosis and adhesions, lateral recess stenosis, disk herniation, and ligamentumflavum hypertrophy. Relative clinical indications for epiduroscopy consist in diagnostic and therapeutic of pain syndromes.

The main indication for epiduroscopy used to be for diagnosis of the sources of pain. Recently, therapeutic is the main indication of the epiduroscopy due to the ability to the treatment of these sites with accuracy. Diagnostically, use of the procedure provides a better view of pathological and anatomical structures and circumstances. Obviously, success of treatment depends on the underlying pathology. Therefore, success or failure of treatment can be used as a measure of the validity of diagnostic parameters obtained through epiduroscopy [10, 12, 13].

As a therapeutic technique, epiduroscopy includes procedures such as direct application of pharmacologic therapy, lysis of scar tissue, adhesions, catheter placement, implantation of stimulation electrodes under direct vision (radio frequency therapy, spinal cord stimulation) and discectomy. Additionally, conscious sedation in patients is administered in order to provide response to stimulated pain-generating areas. Further, epiduroscopy has the potential not only to reduce the incidence of surgery but also to the treatment of post–lumbar surgery syndrome.

Radiculopathy associated with any of the following signs or symptoms is also an indication for epiduroscopy: failed response to epidural steroid injections, filling defects caused by adhesions, post-laminectomy failed back syndrome, and failed conservative back therapy.

The following indications were defined by the consensus committee of the foundation of World Initiative on Spinal Endoscopy (WISE) in 2006 [11]:

To improve diagnosis:

- Diagnosis of clinically relevant epidural pathology, if pain can be attributed to epidural space (spinal canal) structures based on current history, physical examination and supportive present-day laboratory investigations
- Biopsy for histopathological and/or histochemical analysis
- Provocative stimulatory tests (e.g., electrical, light, mechanical)

To provide treatment:

- Irrigation
- Direct application of therapeutic agent
- Direct lysis of adhesions/scar tissue with physical or chemical agents (e.g., mechanical, pharmacological, laser, radio frequency)

As a supportive tool:

- Placing catheter systems (epidural, spinal)
- Implanting stimulation electrodes (spinal cord stimulation)
- As an adjunct in minimally invasive surgery
- Retrieval of foreign bodies
- (Potentially) for post-operative assessment

Contraindications for epiduroscopy

There is a need for confidence in diagnostic to consider contraindications for epiduroscopy, and in particular of the need to differentiate between low back pain of non-spinal origin, such as cognitive affective disorder, and low back pain of psychological origin, for example, compensation psychosis.

The contraindications for epiduroscopy correspond to those for epidural regional anesthesia techniques. The contraindications for regional anesthesia can be listed as skin infections in the area of a cut, hemorrhagic diathesis, anticoagulant therapy, exacerbation of intercurrent illness, flu-like conditions, high cardio-vascular risks, etc.

The contraindications were defined by the consensus committee of the foundation of World Initiative on Spinal Endoscopy (WISE) in 2006 as absolute and relative [11].

The absolute contraindications are stated as follows: psychiatric diseases that potentially interfere with informed consent and/or perception of pain, retinal disease, increased risk for or the presence of elevated intracranial pressure, manifest bowel and bladder, dysfunction and sensory disturbances in S2-S4 area, cerebrovascular disease, advanced systemic diseases, septic or dystrophic skin lesions in the sacral areas (anal fistule, sacral osteomyelitis, etc.), meningeal cysts, meningocele, meningomyelocele, severe respiratory insufficiency (COPD), known allergy for drugs used in the procedure, instable angina, malignancy.

Relative contraindications are as follows: psychiatric diseases that potentially interfere with informed consent and/or perception of pain, inability to lie in a prone position for more than 60 min, severe respiratory insufficiency (COPD), drug or alcohol abuse, etc. [12, 11, 13, 10]

4. Anatomy of epidural space

The main application of epiduroscopy is in relation to the management and treatment of chronic radicular pain. The detailed anatomy of the epidural space and its surrounding bony and ligamentous structures is of great importance for clinicians who perform epiduroscopy. A clear understanding of the relevant anatomy and contents of the space is essential to perform epiduroscopy safely. Epiduroscopic screening with high video-optic quality is enabling displaying of the corresponding morphological structures and visual understanding of this region.

The epidural space is formed between the dural sheath and the spinal canal that extends from the foramen magnum of the skull to the sacral hiatus in combination with the sacrococcygeal ligament. It is bounded superiorly by the fusion of the spinal and periosteal layers of the dura mater at the foramen magnum, and inferiorly by the sacrococcygeal membrane. The epidural space contains the dural sac, the anterior and posterior spinal nerve roots, the extradural venous plexus, spinal arteries, lymphatics, filum terminale and fatty tissue. The anterior and posterior spinal nerve roots are within the dural sac. The dural sac generally ends at the level of the S2 vertebral body and its continuation known as the filum terminale [14].

Anterior or posterior approach to the lumbar epidural space must be used in epidurocopy. Although posterior epiduroscopy can theoretically be performed at any level of the spinal column and through the sacral hiatus, the anterior epiduroscopy must be via caudal approach. Anterior epiduroscopy is the most recent longitudinal approach to the entire lumbar epidural space and provides a significant improvement in the treatment of low-back and leg pain [15].

The sacrum is a wedge-shaped triangular bone at the base of the spinal column that forms from the naturally fused five sacral vertebrae. The sacrum is held in place between the two iliac bones, articulating superiorly with the fifth lumbar vertebra and caudad with the coccyx.

The lamina of the lowest segment of the sacrum is incomplete; therefore, there is a gap which is called the sacral hiatus in the anotomical structure. There are two bony projections that are called the sacral cornua, and the sacrococcygeal ligament which covers this U-shaped space posteriorly. Both of these structures are represent important clinical landmarks when needles are placed into the caudal canal. Penetration of the sacrococcygeal ligament provides direct access to the epidural space of the sacral canal. A superiorly continuation of the sacral canal is the lumbar spinal canal.

Since the spinal cord ends near the level of the second lumbar vertebra, this canal does not carry the spinal cord but contains the epidural venous plexus and is filled with fat, which is subject to an age-related increase in density [16]. Most of these vessels are intensified in the anterior portion of the canal. The advancement of needles or catheters cephalad into the sacral canal can lead to trauma of both the dural sac and epidural vessels.

The epidural space contains prominent amount of epidural fat that distributes along the canal in a predictable pattern allows injected fluid to diffuse through the epidural space and have impact on nerve roots by the absorption of drugs. The fat in the epidural space is soft which surrounds dura mater and protects the neural structures, and facilitates the movement of the dural sac [21].

The spinal dura mater is a strong connective tissue membrane surrounding the cerebral spinal fluid, the spinal cord, the anterior and posterior nerve roots, and spinal ganglia. It extends from the foramen magnum to the sacrum. The dura is being separated by the epidural space so is not attached to the vertebrae. Microscopic view of the dura mater consists of white fibrous and elastic tissues arranged in longitudinal bands or flattened lamellae. Characteristics of dura mater seen on epiduroscopic images are convex, tubular, and grey-white with blood vessels on the surface, giving the appearance of a road map. In epiduroscopy, a fiber-optic endoscope inserted into the sacral hiatus advanced upward into the epidural space. When the epiduroscope advanced in the sacral canal the exact position of dural sac must be ensured via image guidance to prevent dural sac injury because the dural sac terminates at S2 level.

The epidural space contains arteries and veins supplying the spinal cord. The epidural arteries are relatively small and pass through the intervertebral foramina to supply adjacent vertebrae and ligaments. The arteries are located in the lateral epidural space hence not threatened by an advancing needle or epiduroscope. Inside, the spinal canal there is a network of large and valveless veins running along the entire length of the vertebral column. The epidural veins predominantly lie in the anterior epidural space and interconnected one to another to form a venous plexus and ultimately drain into the azygous system of veins. The vertebral plexuses with the veins of bones of the vertebral column form Batson's plexus. The intervertebral veins are responsible for the communication between the vertebral venous plexuses which run through the intervertebral foramina. In the lumbosacral part of the vertebral column, the ventral venous plexus is generally larger than the dorsal plexus. The vertebral venous plexus is subject to distension in case of increased intrathoracic or intra-abdominal pressure because of ascites, pregnancy, large tumors. Thus the venous plexus is thought to be involved in a trauma during epiduroscope placement in the epidural space and increases the risk. [17, 18, 19].

http://dx.doi.org/10.5772/62918

The arteries appear on epiduroscopic images as a thin red thread with pale opaque insulation while veins cannot detectable, and pulsatile flow can be seen [20].

The epidural space communicates with the paravertebral spaces via the intervertebral foramina where major site of action for an epidural located to nerve roots. The nerve supply of the epidural space is via branch from the sinu-vertebral nerves that originate from the rami communicantes. The nerve roots lie in the posterolateral part of the epidural space where they enter and exit the vertebral column at each level in a specific pattern. Nerve roots seen on epiduroscopic images as grey-white tube shape with a vessel running longitudinally down the centre [20, 18].

The lymphatics of the epidural space are present in the region of the dural nerve roots whereas they are absent in the nerve root itself and remove foreign materials from the subarachnoid and epidural spaces [21].

5. Pathological findings of epiduroscopy

Epiduroscopy is the most recent, complete, and effective technique to approach the spine through minimal invasive access means for treating persistent low-back pain.

Spinal pain and radicular pain syndromes are both characterized by pathological and anatomical changes in the epidural space and diagnosed via epiduroscopy such as arachnoiditis, fibrosis, stenosis, nerve root compression.

The epidural space lies between the dura mater and the walls of the vertebral canal, containing fat and small blood vessels. The space is located just outside the dural sac which surrounds the spinal nerve roots and is filled with cerebrospinal fluid.

Epiduroscopic view under traditional white-light endoscopy can give us a better understanding of the pathology. Dura mater appears as either a blue-gray or gray-white exterior with small blood vessels on its surface, epidural fat appears usually yellowish in color, globular, and glistening with small blood vessel on or in it, nerve roots are white tinged with yellow tube shape with a vessel running longitudinally down the center, ligamentum flavum seen as a white and concave tube without vessels.

5.1. Fibrosis

The formation of scar tissue near the nerve root spontaneously or after spine surgery thought to be the potential cause of the pain or radicular symptoms. If it binds the lumbar nerve root with fibrous adhesions that also called epidural fibrosis. Epidural fibrosis also may restrict the flow of medication to the nerve roots and limiting the effectiveness of epidural injections since mechanical deformation of spinal nerve roots and dorsal root ganglions. If the patient suffers from continued or recurrent pain directly after spine surgery epiduroscopic diagnostic imaging technique can often pinpoint the responsible pathology of pain. It was shown that possibility of experience to recurrent radicular pain with an extensive epidural scar is more than less extensive one, and the correlation is statistically significant [22]. None the less a correlation between the degree of epidural fibrosis and the intensity of post-surgical pain was also reported [23, 24]. Epidural fibrosis is diagnosed not only in patients who have had low back surgery but also who have anatomical abnormalities such as stenosis, instabilities and herniated discs without surgery. There are many patients who having pathology with no pain therefore establishing a cause and effect relationship between pathology and pain is low [25]. In the endoscopic image, epidural fibroses appear clear white and are generally avascular.

5.2. Adhesions

Epidural adhesions most commonly occurs as a complication of spinal surgery that are related to inflammatory reactions and result in the entrapment of nerves within dense scar tissue. Beside this can also develop following disc herniation or infection without prior surgery taking place. Morphological changes in the supporting structures of the spine have been identified primarily in the form of epidural adhesions. They limit the pain-free movement and function of structures in the intervertebral foramen and the bony vertebral canal, and prevent direct application of medications to the affected disc and nerve root. Epidural adhesions may or may not involve in the generation of pain therefore should be considered carefully [26, 53]. Adhesions or adhesive areas are easily visible fibrous bands of tissue with epiduroscopy that appear clear to white and often bizarre. Epiduroscopy is used to break down adhesions by infusion of a small amount of saline through the catheter with careful and gentle movement of the catheter.

5.3. Chronic inflammatory processes

The visual function of epiduroscopy can be used to identify chronic inflammatory processes in the epidural space such as epiduritis and radiculitis. Chronic inflammatory condition increases levels of inflammatory mediators at the affected site and results increased pain.

5.4. Radiculitis

Radiculitis is pain that originates from direct pressure on the nerve roots because of inflammation or other irritation of a nerve root at its connection to the spinal column. Disc herniation, osteophytes, thickening of surrounding ligaments, spinal stenosis, damaged intervertebral discs, degeneration of the spine, spondylolisthesis, or scoliosis could be one of the many causes of radiculitis.

Radiculitis symptoms start with radiating pain along the nerve path and usually accompanied with sensations of numbness, tingling, pins, and needles. The other incorporating symptoms of muscle weakness and loss of reflexes also present as the condition progresses. A variety of symptoms of radiculitis can be felt anywhere in the body depending on the location of the affected disc, and nerve root because each area of the body is controlled by nerves exit the spinal column in pairs. For example, cervical nerve root can cause pain and other symptoms through the arms, hands, and fingers, lumbar nerve root can radiate through the leg and into the foot and prompting leg pain and foot pain.

http://dx.doi.org/10.5772/62918

5.5. Epiduritis

Epiduritis is an acute or chronic inflammatory process of epidural structures in the epidural space and on the outer surface of the dura mater of the spinal cord. Epiduroscopically it is characterized with cardinal symptoms such as swelling, redness, and a positive pain provocation test.

5.6. Arachnoiditis

The arachnoid mater is the middle one of the three protective membranes of the central nervous system that surrounds the brain and spinal cord. Inflammation of the arachnoid is called arachnoiditis that subdural processes take place on the caudal fibers and the nerve root sheaths, and characterized by severe burning pain, stinging, numbness, and neurological problems. In the case of arachnoiditis and perineural nerve sheath fibrosis, the spinal dura mater appears thickened and the tissue appeared to have increased vascularization. Arachnoiditis is a complex neuropathic pain disorder with a complex etiology that affects the nerves connecting to the lower back and legs. Adhesive arachnoiditis is most commonly present with associated epidural fibrosis whereas epidural fibrosis can occur alone. Arachnoiditis is most frequently seen in patients who have undergone multiple surgical procedures.

5.7. Xanthosis

Xanthosis is a yellowish degeneration with yellowish pigmentation which could be observed in the spinal epidural space in the literature by Heavner et al. [27]. This epiduroscopy finding in the peridural tissue adjacent to blood vessels at the left L5-S1 intervertebral foramen associated with radiculopathy. They administered treatment with the same equipment and gained satisfactory reduction in the radicular pain with the treatment outcome. Thus, called as a novo epiduroscopy finding.

5.8. Ligamentum flavum hypertrophy

Hypertrophy of the ligamentum flavum is a pathologic condition due to fibrosis and scar tissue formation that contribute to cord compression radiculopathy. Hypertrophy of the ligamentum flavum can be rarely encountered in the lumbar region however more common in cervical and thoracic regions. Hypertrophy of the ligamentum flavum is usually involved in the pathogenesis of spinal stenosis which can cause loss of disc height, reduce the diameter of the spinal canal and compress the dural sac and nerve roots. A multilevel detailed examination of the epidural space is now possible with epiduroscopy and directly observation of hypertrophied ligamentum flavum can be satisfactorily achieved [28, 29].

5.9. Cysts in the spinal canal

The patients may suffer from recurrent pain and/or troublesome new symptoms such as failed back surgery syndrome after surgical treatment. Some cyst types may also be present in the different levels of the spinal canal such as synovial cyst of a lumbar facet joint, often cause spinal compression and radicular pain. Even if these cysts can be visualized in epiduroscopic imaging, due to the packed up anatomy and the inflamed cyst being not easily identified from adjacent structures confirmation of the diagnosis with fluoroscopy, MRI or CT may be necessary to assess the contents of spinal canal [30]. Minimally invasive technique such as cyst rupture by epiduroscopy has the potential for fenestration of cyst either post-operative or not.

Jin et al. successfully removed a lumbar facet joint cyst at L4/5 level by epiduroscopy. Epiduroscopy usage as a support to diagnose and therapy of the cyst that results compression on the radicular nerve would be favorably an alternative technique over conventional surgery in the future [31].

6. Technique of epiduroscopy

Before the epiduroscopy process, the patient's history should be reviewed as expeditiously as possible and a comprehensive physical exam should be carried out. Detailed preoperative knowledge of the patient's neurological assessment is necessary to recognize the post-operative neurological complications. The specialized nerve tests such as EMG, NCV and SSEP to investigate the functioning of the nervous system, and imaging studies like CT scans or MRI scans should be completed in the preoperative setting. The skeletal structures of the sacrum, the level of termination and position of the bottom of the dural sac particularly on T2-weighted MRI, the evaluation of the anterior and posterior epidural spaces should be performed previously.

Epidural bleeding during epiduroscopy constitute extremely rare, however, taking conventional precautions to prevent is substantial. NSAIDs use should be stopped 24 h before and aspirin should be stopped 3–4 days before procedure in the perioperative period. It is also generally recommended to stop any oral anticoagulant before open surgery. In addition to complete blood count (CBC) that also called hemogram, an evaluation of basic coagulation

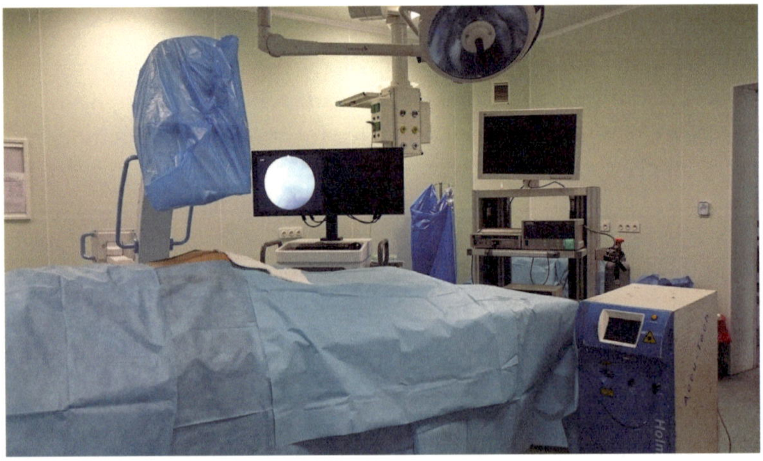

Figure 1. Optimum design of the operating room at which the epiduroscopy takes place.

parameters should be ordered for prothrombin time (PT) with a partial thromboplastin time (PTT), and the international normalized ratio (INR) calculation based on results of PT to monitor individuals in the perioperative period. The operating room is equipped with a fluoroscopy table, C-armed scopy device, holmium laser, light source, and imaging device (**Figures 1–3**).

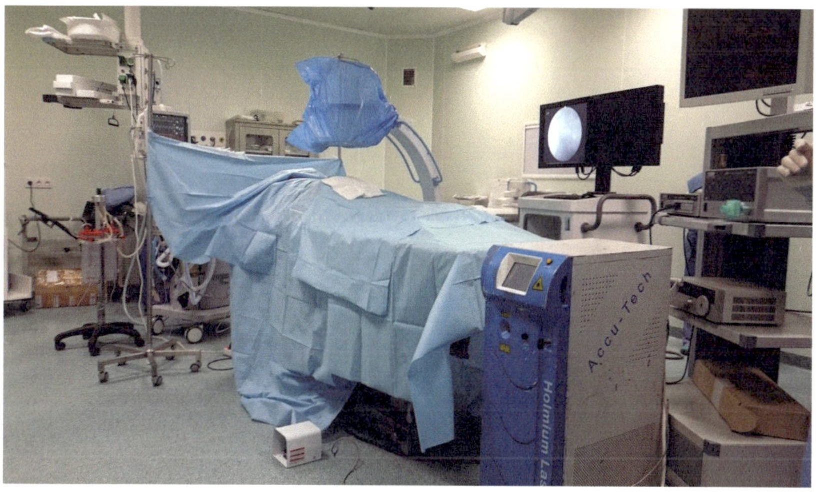

Figure 2. Anesthesia device in front of the operating table.

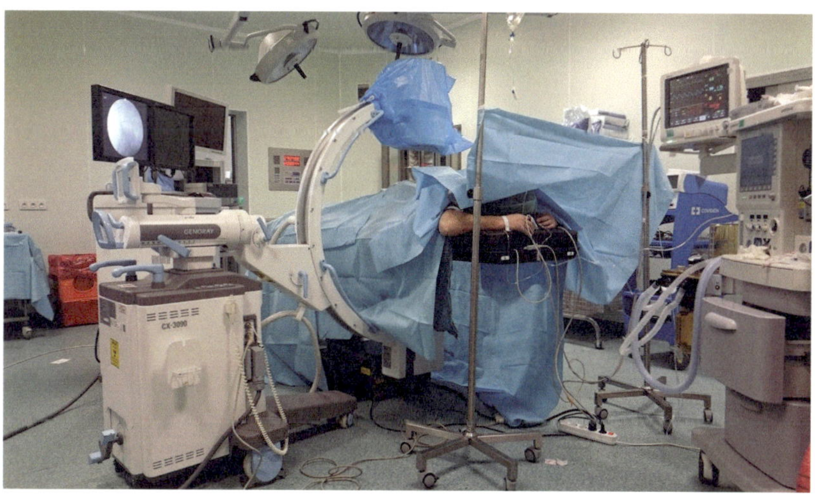

Figure 3. C-armed scope and video monitoring system to the right of operating table, Holmium laser device and tradle close to applicator.

Perioperative antibiotic prophylaxis therapy in general administration of ceftriaxone 1 g intravenously should be given within 1 h before epiduroscopy. The patient is admitted to the operation room and placed in the prone position on the fluoroscopy table with a pillow under the abdomen to correct the lumbar lordosis.

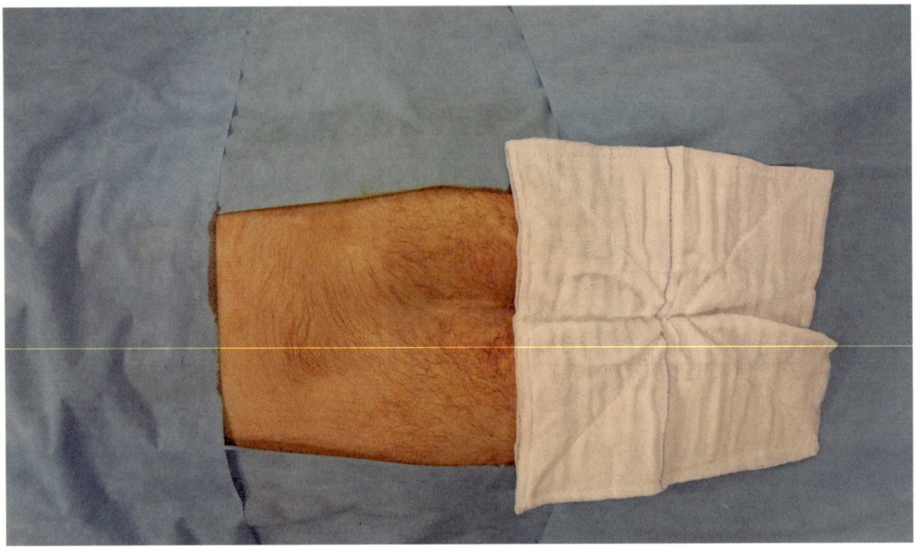

Figure 4. After setting aseptic conditions, sterile dressing gets covered over procedure area.

The practice of aseptic technique is maintained and patient and fluoroscopy are covered the sterile dressing (**Figure 4**). Intravenous 2 mg midazolam and 50 mcg fentanyl is administered for performing the procedure under conscious sedation.

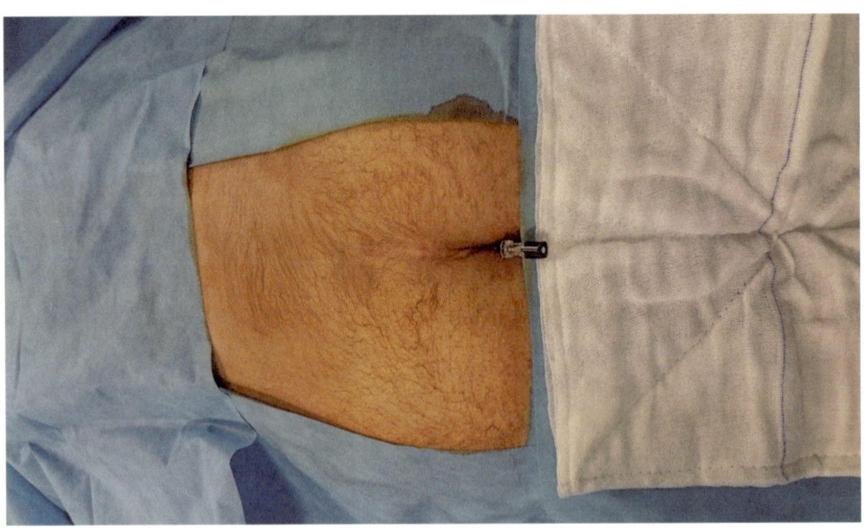

Figure 5. Insertion of 22G spinal needle passing through sacral hiatus.

http://dx.doi.org/10.5772/62918

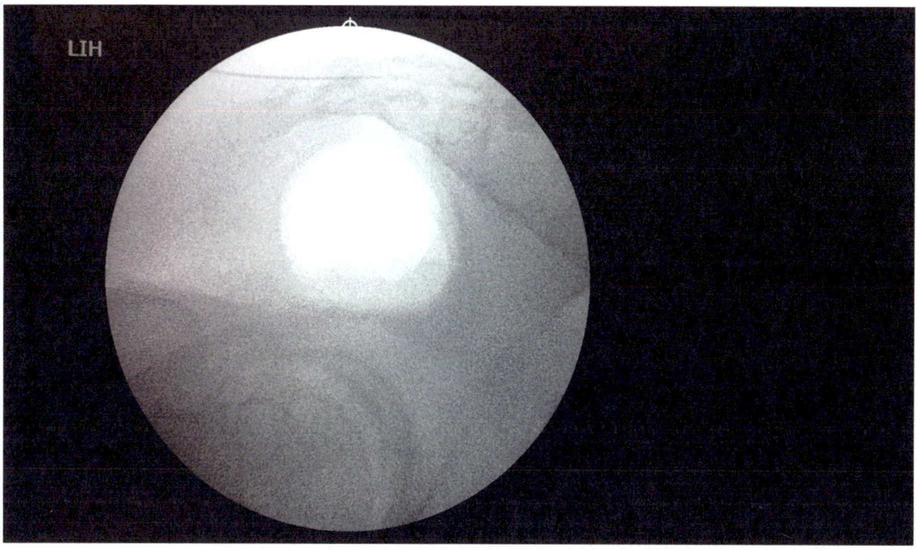

Figure 6. Fluoroscopy image of 22G spinal needle after passing through sacral hiatus.

Under C-arm (fluoroscope) lateral image guidance, intradermal, and subdermal infiltration of local anesthetic is injected by a 22G spinal needle, then 8–10 mL 1% lidocaine injection is administered to epidural space by passing through the sacral hiatus (**Figures 5** and **6**). This will greatly reduce the abnormal pain and pressure feeling of patient during advancing the trocar through the narrow caudal canal, will prevent in vivo motion in patient and there will be no need to increase the sedation of prone-positioned patient so that facilitates ease of application for clinician.

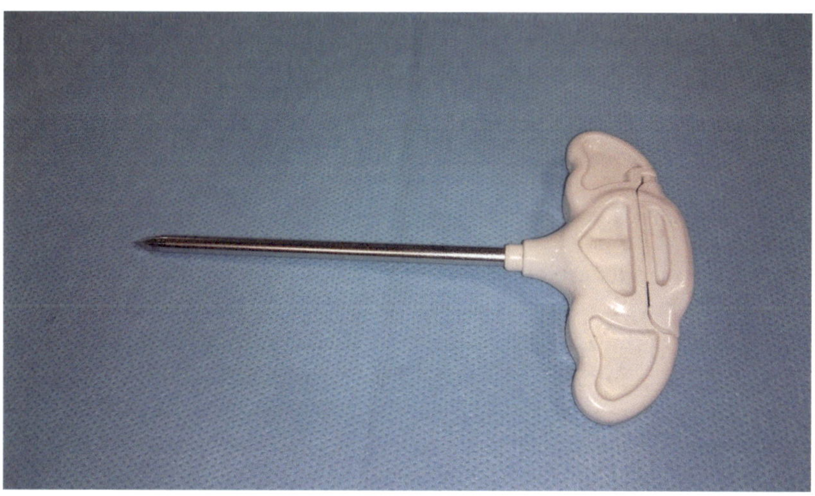

Figure 7. 4.2 mm outer diameter and 3.5 mm inner diameter ranged trocar.

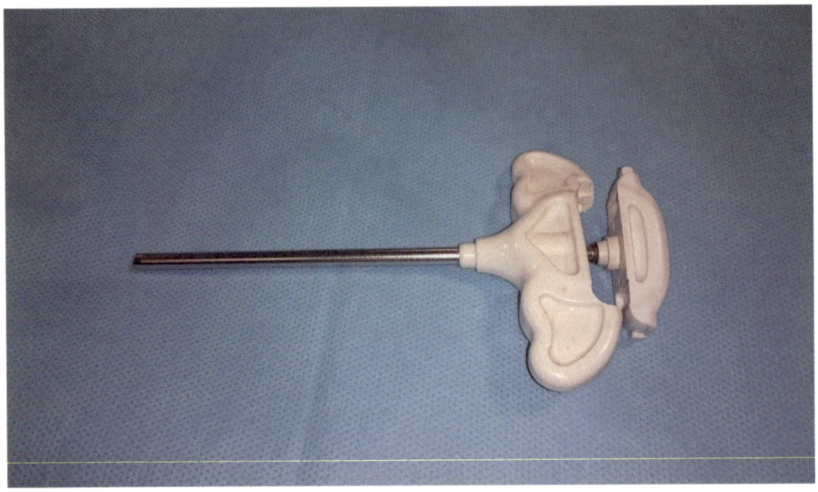

Figure 8. Image of trocar after its stilette is removed.

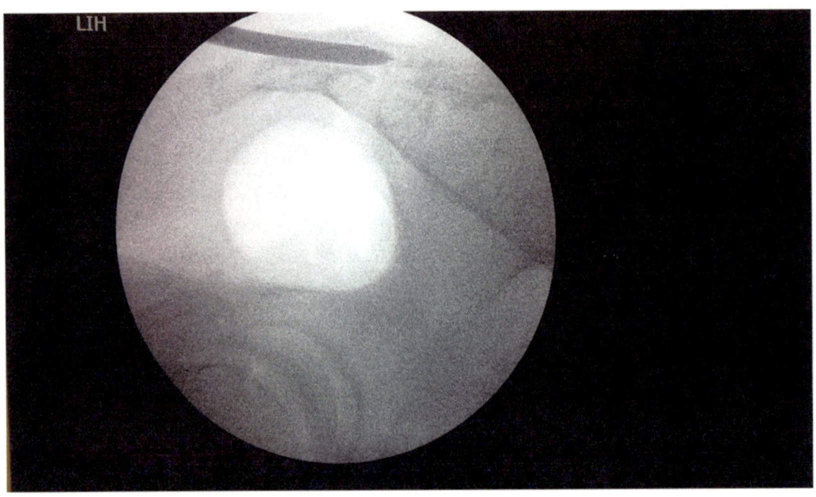

Figure 9. The lateral fluoroscopic image of trocar in the caudal epidural space after passing through sacral hiatus.

Lateral intradermal and subdermal incision of 0.5 cm is made in the skin with No. 11 sharp disposable scalpel where 22G spinal needle introduced. If you notice some bleeding from the incision simply apply firm pressure to the area with surgical gauze. The trocar is, outer diameter 4.2 mm and inner diameter 3.5 mm, and then advanced through sacral hiatus at the skin incision point with C-armed scopy guidance (**Figures 7–9**). There is a slight loss of resistance as the trocar enters the caudal canal. Repeat antero-posterior (AP) images will be taken during the trocar advancement and will assure that the trocar direction does not stray from midline. AP image confirmation of proper placement of the trocar in the mid-line of sacral foramina will verify its position within the same line of pubic symphysis. The C-armed scopy is rotated in a lateral direction once trocar is held on the posterior to dural sac, where termination and position of the bottom of the dural sac was determined previously on MRI, and the central stylet of the trocar is pulled out.

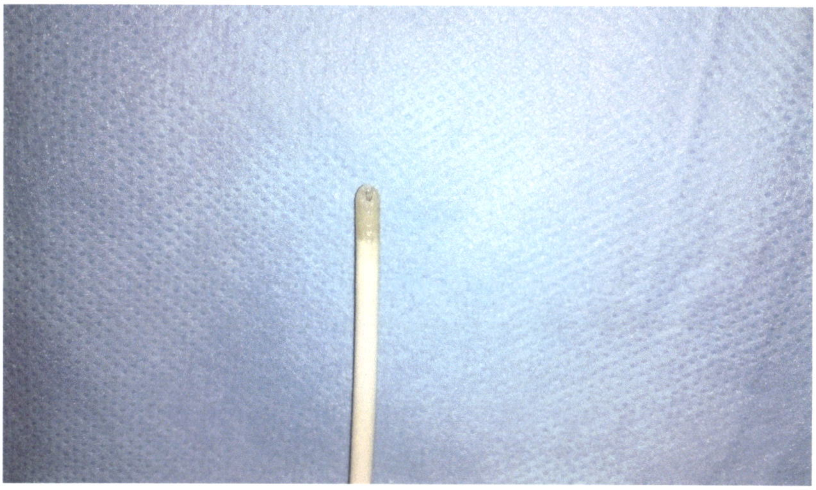

Figure 10. Image of epiduroscope catheter tip.

Spinaut-V® epiduroscopy catheter is 33 cm in length and outer diameter 3.2 mm in width. The catheter has two working channel in 1.2 mm diameter where one is maintained on the top and the other is at the bottom of device. (**Figure 10**). The top canal is for using a high resolution fiber optic camera, and the bottom canal is for using a laser probe or biopsy forceps that can ablate a herniated disc or epidural scar tissue (**Figures 11** and **12**). The device has an ergonomic design for handling the epiduroscope. There is a controller gear on both sides of catheter to steer the catheter in 2-way directions (right or left). There is a dual port on the back of controller gear look like a dual exhaust. (**Figure 13**). On the left input, the canal allows insertion of camera and physiological saline solution administration at the same time to give a clear view of the inside of the epidural space during the procedure (**Figure 14**). Extension tubing for extension line is connected to the left input and attached to physiological saline bag 150 mL via a 3-way stop-cock. A 20-mL injector is also connected to the 3-way stop-cock. Physiological saline solution is injected either by exerting a light pressure on the injector or slow infusion. In the right input; there is a tube outlet that allows suction of blood or other given solutions. Non-ionic radio-opaque material is preferred to be administered through the right canal because it is highly dense and can stick to camera that results blurred image. This happens more frequently when it is administered through left canal. Additionally; injecting physiological saline along with radio-opaque material will pull away the material away from the camera. The best way of avoiding the blurred image and obtaining good visualization of the epidural space is passing camera through the epiduroscope after application of the initial epidurography.

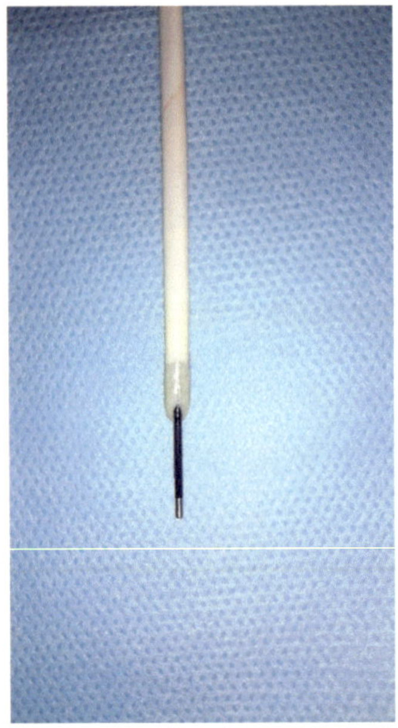

Figure 11. Camera and laser probe from superior and lateral taken from epiduroscope catheter tip.

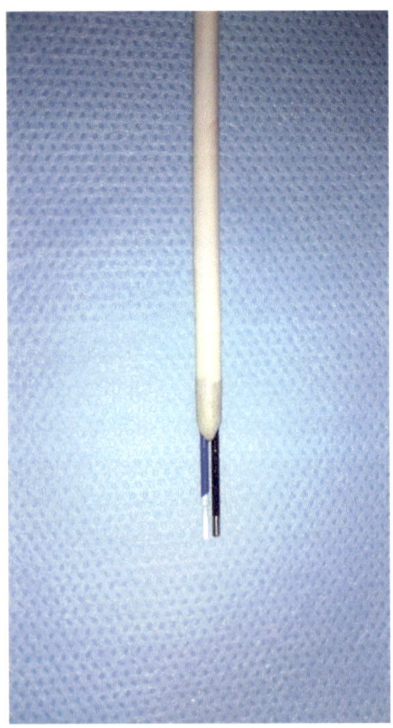

Figure 12. Laser probe and camera are superposed in the upper shooting.

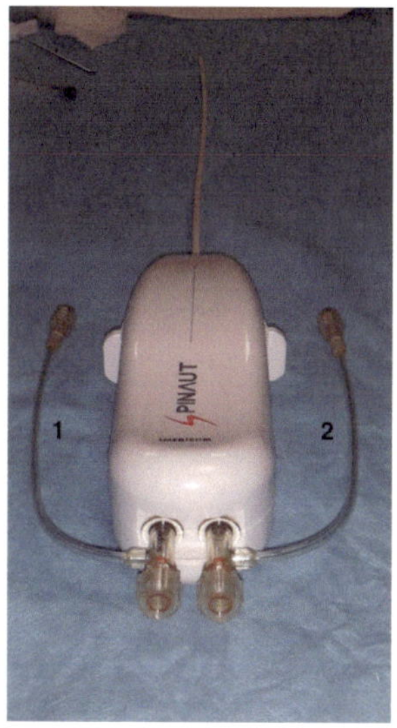

Figure 13. Fiberoptic camera advances from the left input (1), laser probe advances from the right input (2).

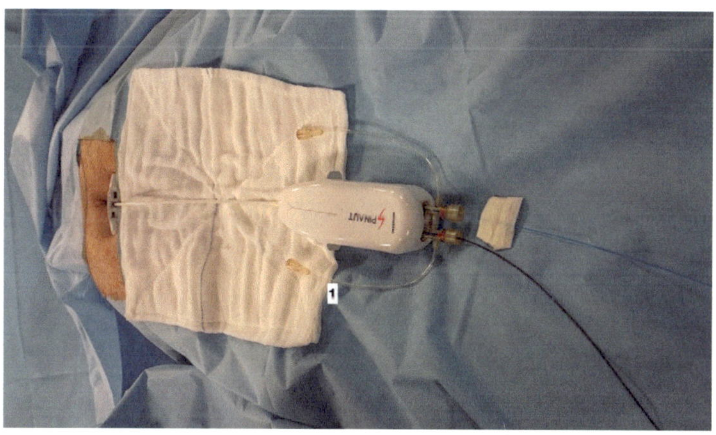

Figure 14. Physiologic saline line (1).

In the case of access to posterior epidural space, epiduroscopy is passed through the trocar and advanced to S1 vertebra level with guidance of C-armed scopy. After the epiduroscopy is placed, 10 mL of radio-opaque material is injected for epidurography. The monitoring of epidural space is started after re-evaluating the clinical condition of patient, MRI, and epidurography results.

The epiduroscope is rotated 90° laterally to gain access into the anterior epidural space and advanced through trocar under the guidance of C-armed scopy lateral imaging. While attempting to introduce epiduroscopy into the anterior epidural space rotating the scope too much may lead folding of the catheter tip, an abrupt turn of epiduroscope to the left or right that cause sensation of pain may lead patient movement and induce loss of the position of the patient. Following the access into the anterior epidural space, epiduroscope is returned to original neutral position.

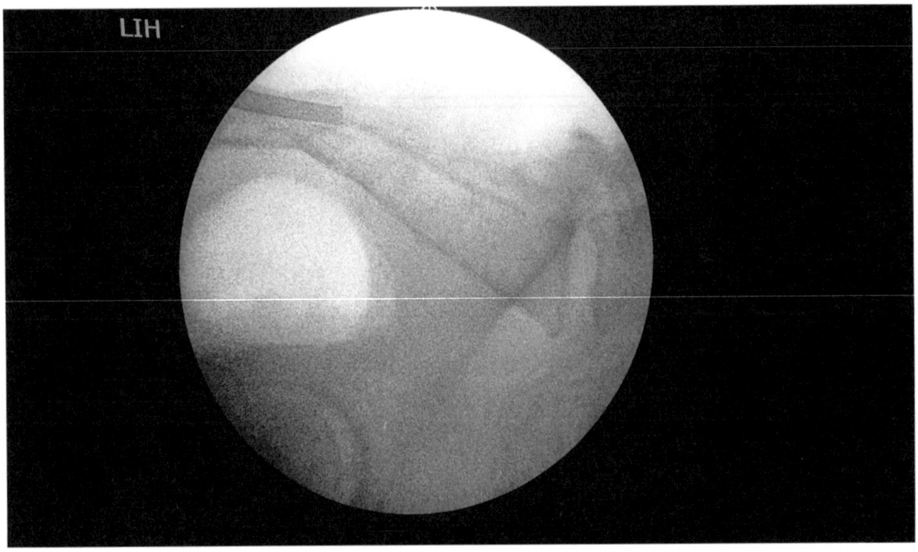

Figure 15. The lateral fluroscopic image of epiduroscope tip at S1 level.

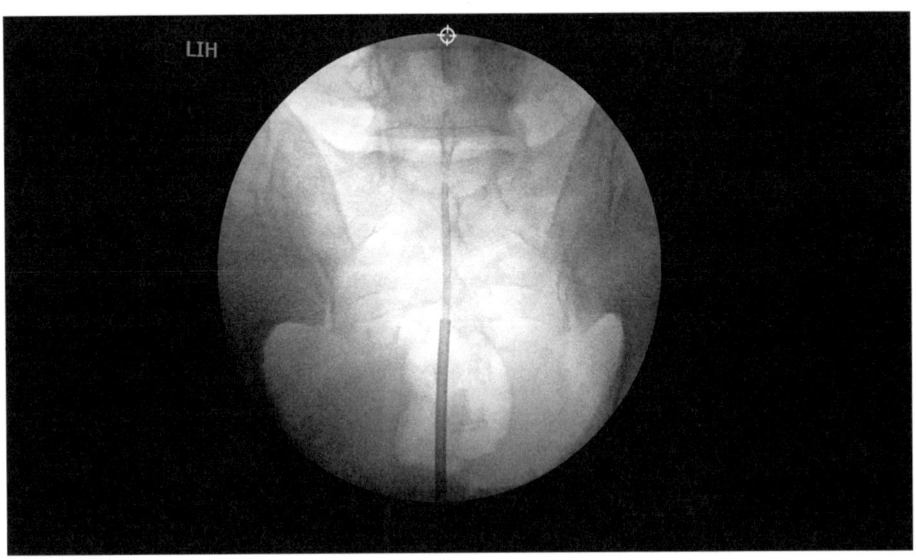

Figure 16. The AP fluroscopic image of epiduroscope tip at S1 level.

Once epiduroscope inserted into the anterior epidural space, the tip of the epiduroscope is introduced to the level of S1 (**Figures 15** and **16**). Initial epidurography is done at the same time to detect disc herniation or obstruction level, and compared to MRI and clinical findings. The bulging at targeted disc level is easily seen due to obstruction to the flow of the injected radio-opaque material towards to cephal. By use of the AP fluoroscopy position, the end-plates of targeted levels are straightened. The fiberoptic camera with light is connected to epiduroscope under sterile conditions and advanced through the left input until the epiduroscopic end point. The camera that the light source system controlled and white balanced prior to procedure to assure accurate tissue color is turned on. Injection of physiological saline through the catheter placed into the epidural space would keep distend the epidural space and keep clear the camera for a good view. The piston of physiological saline containing injector is slightly pushed (0.15–0.20 mL/s). The amount of given hidration must be tightly monitorized. The fiberoptic camera shouldnot get pass the end point of epiduroscope because the vision from the camera is designed to fit the opening of epiduroscope to point upwards. This way we obtain a crescent shaped edge beneath the monitorized view and use this as a kind of compass. Keeping the crescent edge at the bottom part of the image allows us proper orientation in the anterior epidural canal. While in the anterior epidural canal, as we get the crescent at the bottom the dura will be appear at the upper side of the image on the screen. As we are able to monitor both dura and lumbar disk at the same time, laser probe that is introduced into respective input canal does not harm the dura and placed in the targeted disk.

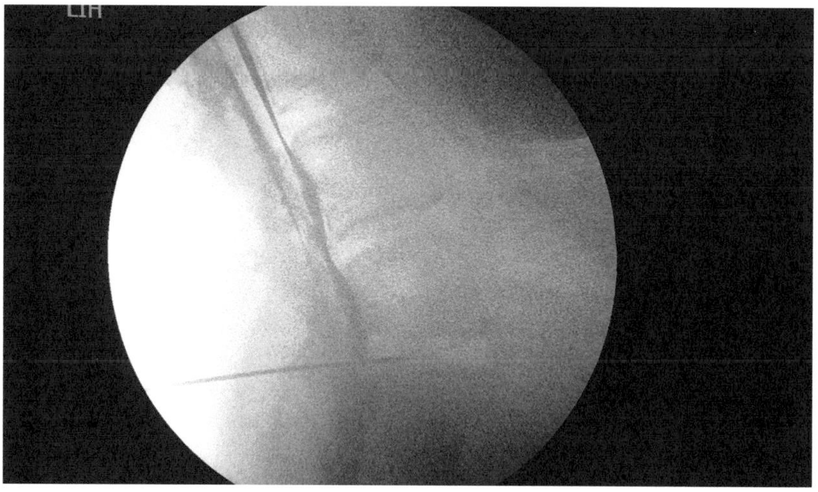

Figure 17. The lateral fluoroscopic image of upward passing of radio-opac material through anterior and posterior openings.

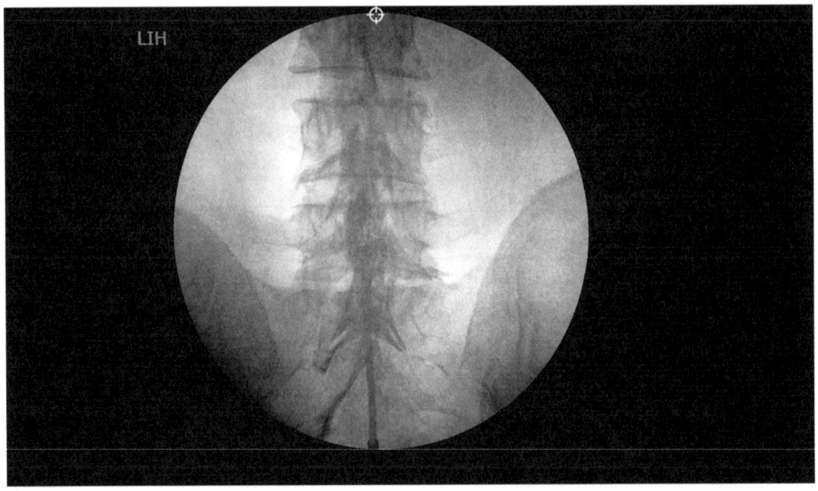

Figure 18. The final AP epidurography.

Before the termination of procedure, a final epidurography is performed to assess the efficiency of epiduroscopy (**Figures 17** and **18**). If the patient did not diagnosed with diabetes mellitus and the dura was not perforated, 80 mg of methyl prednisolone and 10–15 mg of bupivacaine in 5 mL total volume would be injected and the trocar along with the epiduroscopy catheter is removed.

When the procedure is over, a single suture for skin closure is applied and wound dressing is completed. The patient is admitted to post-op care unit and evaluated. If no abnormality is observed the patient is discharged to the ward. The patient is immobilized for 3–4 h. Especially in patients with disc herniation is advised to use steel corset while mobilizing. The pain in the intervention point and headache are the most common complications of an epidural procedure. To manage this, intravenous hydration treatment and intravenous 1 gr of paracetamol are sufficient. If there is no problem in their general clinic condition, patients can be discharged at same day or can be admitted to the ward for one night then discharged the day after the procedure with antibiotics and NSAIDs prescription. Because of the administration of steroids to epidural region, 7–10 days of salt-free diet is reasonable. Perineal care is advised cleaning of the perineum from dorsal to front without contacting the intervention point after defecation/urination is advised. Patients are permitted to take their first shower 1–2 days after the epiduroscopy

7. Therapeutic anterior epiduroscopy

Epiduroscopy has been introduced as a new technique for treatment of chronic low back pain (LBP) syndromes or herniated disks. The clinical effectiveness and cost-effectiveness of epiduroscopy have been described in multiple prospective and retrospective studies although the underlying mechanisms have not been fully investigated.

The procedures used for determination of the pathology in chronic low back pain often have difficulty in making an accurate diagnosis. However, epidural endoscope allows visualization of the epidural space to potentially identify the reason of LBP, therefore, to address these problems attention has been drawn to epiduroscopy as a tool for an accurate diagnosis. In addition to more accurate diagnosis, usage as a therapy of any adhesion or inflammation, compression on the radicular nerve therein, and inject medications into the lesions.

7.1. Epiduroscopic laser discectomy

Disc decompression is typically performed both surgically and non-surgically to reduce pressure on the nerve root by removing disc nucleus while preserving disc strength with a high success rate, [1, 2] and low complication rate [32, 33].

Technological innovations in the treatment of disc decompressions has improved the ability to treat pathology effectively through anterior epiduroscopy that requires only local anesthetic and conscious sedation (leading to reduced risk of accidental nerve damage), overcomes the possible complications of surgery and general anesthesia.

Recently, epiduroscopic laser neural decompression (ELND) as another minimal invasive technique have been introduced for chronic low back pain and radicular pain that cannot be solved by other non-invasive conservative treatments, including the epidural steroid injection [34]. In spite of surgery is often considered as the next step in treating continuous chronic low back pain, it has potential risks of post–lumbar surgery syndrome that is difficult to manage. The incidence of post–lumbar surgery syndrome after back surgery ranges from 5 to 50% [35].

Laser is a source of monochromatic, coherent and unidirectional light that used in many fields of medicine with diagnostic and therapeutic purposes. Disc and neural decompression, rechanneling stenoses caused by adhesions are examples of the use of laser and expands the range of possibilities for epiduroscopy. Researches involving lasers have been conducted on the usefulness of epiduroscope for the patients with the post–lumbar surgery syndrome. Epiduroscopic laser application allows treatment of low back pain and radicular pain caused by herniated lumbar disc, adhesions or fibrosis in the epidural space depending on the particular pathological and anatomical circumstances [36, 37].

In the treatment of patients with chronic refractory low back pain a two working channel system of video guided catheter and subsequent application of an optical laser fiber is established. As with the existing epiduroscopic adhesiolysis, epiduroscopic laser neural decompression (ELND) also provides non-invasiveness, short operating time, elimination of the risks of general anesthesia, communication with the patient during the procedure, and short recovery time. ELND offers a variety of additional benefits that direct treatment of the origin of pathology by reducing the volume of the herniated disc in the affected area, direct removal of severely adhered areas with the laser, no occurrence of laser-related oedema or adhesions.

However, an excellent visual control is compulsory for the use of laser where the endoscope with the flexible tip makes possible advancement fine navigation of the relatively rigid laser fiber. Further visual control has to assured and saline infusion has to be started prior to the laser activation.

Because of the risks of heat damage to the nerve roots induced by laser disc decompression, treatment of adhesions near the nerve root should be avoided. Epiduroscopic laser neural decompression can easily remove painful adhesions in the area of the nerve root that cannot mobilized by mechanical movement of the tip of the epiduroscope.

If motor nerve paralysis occurs due to thermal damage of nerve roots during the laser treatment as a complication, the procedure must be aborted immediately. Other complications those need particular caution have been reported as local sensory impairment, fiber breakage, and discitis during the laser procedure [38].

8. Complications

In spite of epiduroscopy is a safe technique as a minimal invasive procedure to reduce post-operative complications, the rates of complications will increase commensurate with its increasing usage.

Complications arising during epidurocsopy therapy are mainly reported as headache, cervicodynia, convulsions, dura tear, neurologic damage, visual impairment, infection, general back complaints, vomiting, meningitis, radicular radiating pain, bladder, dizziness, hypoacousia, and rectal disorders.

According to the literature, complications related to epiduroscopy are generally caused by puncture trauma, accidental dural injury, puncture of an epidural blood vessel or epidural bleeding, changes in the epidural pressure caused by saline infusion [39, 40, 42, 45, 49, 50]. The knowledge on the complications and accidental symptoms, using proper epiduroscopic equipment and ensuring optimal vision accompanied with sufficient experience in using the epiduroscopic technique can help prevention from complications.

Post–dural puncture headache are reported relatively frequently during epiduroscopy when attempting to carry out placement of the epiduroscopic catheter or from accidental perforation of the dura as a result of perforation of the spinal dura mater and attributed to a rapid loss of cerebrospinal fluid.

The dural perforation is not a serious complication unless the accidental dural perforation is not recognized and is not responded to, otherwise, spontaneous closure of the perforated site has also observed. Epidural blood patches are reliable in order to treat the patients' headache due to dural perforation during epiduroscopy within a short time [41, 43, 44, 47, 48].

It is reported by Gill and Heavner [51] that a sudden increase in epidural pressure due to the epidural infusion causes compression of the optic nerve and compression of the vessels that results to a rupture and in turn to retinal haemorrhage.

Another clinically relevant complication described by Mizuno et al. [46] in which encephalopathy and rhabdomyolysis was induced by the administration of the contrast agent iotrolan during epiduroscopy.

Our experience has also shown that the amount of liquids delivered to the spinal canal should be calculated precisely during implementation of the epiduroscopy procedure, and infusion rate of drug or radiopaque substances should be at a low speed to avoid from complications. When saline fluid was infused too quickly this leaded to hypertension, decreased oxygen saturation, respiratory arrest, and loss of consciousness where epiduroscopy was immediately terminated [52].

The incidence of complications is inversely proportional to professional skills of practitioner and the number of years of experience. It should be bear in mind, there are risks associated with medical procedures in the spinal region, even when it is performed properly and conscientiously.

Author details

Havva Sayhan and Serbulent Gokhan Beyaz*

*Address all correspondence to: sgbeyaz@gmail.com

Faculty of Medicine, Sakarya University, Sakarya, Turkey

References

[1] Heavner J, Chokhavatia S, Kizelshteyn G. Percutaneous evaluation of the epidural and subarachnoid space with a flexible fiberscope. Reg Anesth. 1991;15(1):85.

[2] Richter EO, Abramova MV, Cantu F, DeAndres J, Lierz P, Manchiaro PL, Van Buyten JP, Kim JD, Jang JH, Jung GH, Kim JY, Jang S, Salgado H, Salgado P, Alo KM. Anterior epiduroscopic neural decompression: eight-center experience in 154 patients. Eur J Pain Suppl. 2011;5(2):401–407.

[3] Burman M. Myeloscopy or the direct visualisation of the spinal canal and its contents. J Bone Joint Surg. 1931;13:695–696.

[4] Pool J. Myeloscopy: intraspinal endoscopy. Surgery. 1942;11:169–182.

[5] Hirschowitz BI, Curtiss LE, Peters CW, Pollard HM. Demonstration of a new gastroscope, the fiberscope. Gastroenterology. 1958;35(1):discussion 51–3.

[6] Ooi Y, Morisaki N. Intrathecal lumbar endoscope. Clin Orthop Surg (Japan). 1969;4:295–297.

[7] Saberski LR, Kitahata LM. Direct visualization of the lumbosacral epidural space through the sacral hiatus. Anesth Analg. 1995;80:839–840.

[8] Leu HF, Hauser RK, Schreiber A. Lumbar percutaneous endoscopic interbody fusion. Clin Orthop Relat Res. 1997;337:58–63.

[9] Schutze G, Kurtse G, Grol O, Enns E. Endoscopic method for the diagnosis and treatment of spinal pain syndromes. Anesteziol Reanimatol. 1996;4:62–64.

[10] Ruetten S, Meyer O, Godolias G. Endoscopic surgery of the lumbar epidural space (epiduroscopy): results of therapeutic intervention in 93 patients. Minim Invasive Neurosurg. 2003;46(1):1–4.

[11] Beltrutti D, Groen GJ, Lloyd Saberski L, Kiesling AS, Schutze G, Weber G. Epiduroscopy Consensus Decision March, 2006. In: World Initiative on Spinal Endoscopy (WISE) Consensus Conference; 3–4 March; Graz (Austria). Austria, 2006.

[12] Avellanal M, Reganon GD, Orts A, Montero LG, Ares JA.. Epiduroscopy: Complications and troubleshooting. Tech Reg Anesth Pain Manage. 2014;1(8):35–39.

[13] Bosscher HA, Heavner JE. Lumbosacral epiduroscopy findings predict treatment outcome. Pain Pract. 2014;14(6):506–14.

[14] Westbrook JL. Anatomy of the epidural space. Anaesth Intensive Care Med. 2012;13(11):551–554.

[15] Richter E, Abramova M, Mussell J. Current trends in minimally invasive spinal surgery. J Neurosurg Rev. 2011;1(1):1–13.

[16] Schütze G. Epiduroscopy Spinal Endoscopy. 1st ed. Heidelberg: Springer Medizin Verlag; 2008. 156 p.

[17] Ellis H. The anatomy of the epidural space. Anaesth Intensive Care Med. 2009;10(11): 533–35.

[18] Brockway M. Focus on: central neural blockade anatomy of the epidural space. Curr Anaesth Crit Care. 1999;10:118–122.

[19] Richardson J, Groen GJ. Applied epidural anatomy continuing education in anaesthesia. Contin Educ Anaesth Crit Care Pain 2005;5(3): 98–100

[20] Lee PB, Kim SO, Kim YC. Epiduroscopic Adhesiolysis. In: Kim DH, editor. Minimally Invasive Percutaneous Spinal Techniques. 1st ed. Elsevier; 2011.

[21] Ogan SF. Anatomy and Clinical Importance of the Epidural Space. In: Ogan SF, editor. Epidural Analgesia—Current Views and Approaches. 1st ed. Crotia: Intech; 2012. pp. 1–13.

[22] Maroon JC, Abla A, Bost J. Association between peridural scar and persistent low back pain after lumbar discectomy. Neurol Res. 1999;21 (1):S43–620.

[23] Almeida DB, Prandini MN, Awamura Y, Vitola ML, Simião MP, Milano JB, Bordignon KC, Ache MP, Ramina R. Outcome following lumbar disc surgery: the role of fibrosis. Acta Neurochir. 2008;150(11):1167–1176.

[24] Rönnberg K,Lind B, Zoega B, Göthlin GG, Halldin K, Gellerstedt M, Brisby H. Peridural scar and its relation to clinical outcome: a randomised study on surgically treated lumbar disc herniation patients. Eur Spine J. 2008;17(12):1714–1720.

[25] Jarvik JG, Deyo RA. Diagnostic evaluation of low back pain with emphasis on imaging. Ann Intern Med. 2002;137(7):586–597.

[26] Quintero G, Hugo V, Pachano C, Francisco E. Preventing adhesions in obstetric and gynecologic surgical procedures. Rev Obstet Gynecol. 2009;2(1):38–45.

[27] Heavner JE, Bosscher H, Dunn D, Lehman T. Xanthosis in the spinal epidural space an epiduroscopy finding. Pain Practice. 2004;4(1):39–41.

[28] Sairyo K, Biyani A, Goel VK, Leaman DW, Booth R Jr, Thomas J, Ebraheim NA, Cowgill IA, Mohan SE. Lumbar ligamentum flavum hypertrophy is due to accumulation of inflammation-related scar tissue. Spine (Phila Pa 1976). 2007;32(11):E340–7.

[29] Krasuski P, Poniecka AW, Gal E, Walid A, Truonga A, Harte AML. Epiduroscopy: review of technique and results. Pain Clin. 2001;13(1):71–76.

[30] Jin HS, Bae JY, In CB, Choi EJ, Lee PB, Oct FS. Epiduroscopic removal of a lumbar facet joint cyst. Korean J Pain. 2015;28(4):275–279.

[31] Hoshino Y, Sumitani M, Kusakabe Y, Sato K, Tomioka T, Ogawa M, Sekiyama H, Yamada Y. Successful treatment of spinal canal cystic lesion with the epiduroscopy: a case report. J Jpn Soc Pain Clin. 2012;19 (2):98–102.

[32] Alò KM, Wright RE, Sutcliffe J, Brandt SA. Percutaneous lumbar discectomy: one-year follow-up in an initial cohort of 50 consecutive patients with chronic radicular pain. Pain Pract. 2005;5(2):116–123.

[33] Carragee EJ, Han MY, Yang B, Kim DH, Kraemer H, Billys J. Activity restrictions after posterior lumbar discectomy: a prospective study of outcomes in 152 cases with no postoperative restrictions. Spine. 1999;24(22):2346–2351.

[34] Jo DH, Yang HJ. The survey of the patient received the epiduroscopic laser neural decompression. Korean J Pain. 2013;26:27–31.

[35] Takeshima N, Miyakawa H, Okuda K, Hattori S, Hagiwara S, Takatani J, Noguchi T. Evaluation of the therapeutic results of epiduroscopic adhesiolysis for failed back surgery syndrome. Br J Anaesth. 2009;102:400–407.

[36] Ruetten S, Meyer O, Godolias G. Epiduroscopic diagnosis and treatment of epidural adhesions in chronic back pain syndrome of patients with previous surgical treatment: first results of 31 interventions. Z Orthop Ihre Grenzgeb. 2002;140(2):171–175.

[37] Hayek SM, Helm S, Benyamin RM, Singh V, Bryce DA, Smith HS. Effectiveness of spinal endoscopic adhesiolysis in post lumbar surgery syndrome: a systematic review. Pain Phys. 2009;12(2):419–435.

[38] Ahn JS. Laser decompression. J Korean Soc Spine Surg. 2000;7:318–321.

[39] Racz GB, Heavner JE, Trescot A. Percutaneous lysis of epidural adhesions—Evidence for safety and efficacy. Pain Pract. 2008;8(4):277–286.

[40] Talu GK, Erdine S. Complications of epidural neuroplasty: a retrospective evaluation. Neuromodulation. 2003;6(4):237–247.

[41] Perkins WJ, David DH, Huntoon MA, Horlocker TT. A retained Racz catheter fragment after epidural neurolysis: implications during magnetic resonance imaging. Anesth Analg. 2003;96(6):1717–1719.

[42] Richter H. Is the so-called epidural neuroplasty (Racz catheter) a harmless procedure? In: Neurochirurgie DGf, ed. Deutsche Gesellschaft Fur Neurochirurgie. Strasbourg, Germany: Deutsche Gesellschaft fur Neurochirurgie; 2005.

[43] Wagner KJ, Sprenger T, Pecho C, Kochs EF, Tölle TR, Berthele A, Gerdesmeyer L. Risks and complications of epidural neurolysis—a review with case report. Anesthesiol Intensmed Notfallmed Schmerzther. 2006;41(4):213–222.

[44] Moschos MM, Rouvas A, Papaspirou A, Apostolopoulos M. Acute visual loss and intraocular hemorrhages associated with endoscopic spinal surgery. Clin Ophthalmol. 2008;2(4):937–939.

[45] Heavner J, Wyatt DE, Bosscher H. Lumbosacral epiduroscopy complicated by intravascular injection. Anesthesiology. 2007;107(2):347–350.

[46] Mizuno J, Gauss T, Suzuki M, Hayashida M, Arita H, Hanaoka K. Encephalophaty and rhabdomyolysis induced by iotrolan during epiduroscopy. Can J Anaesth. 2007;54(1): 49–53.

[47] Komiya K, Igarashi T, Suzuki H, Hirabayashi Y, Waechter J, Seo N. In vitro study of patient's and physician's radiation exposure in the performance of epiduroscopy. Reg Anesth Pain Med. 2008;33(2):98–101.

[48] Heavner JE, Bosscher H. Epiduroscopy and radiation exposure. Reg Anesth Pain Med. 2009;34(1):79.

[49] Avellanala M, Diaz-Reganona G, Ortsa A, Gonzalez-Monteroa L, Aresc JA. Epiduroscopy complications and troubleshooting. Techniques in Regional Anesthesia and Pain Management. 2014;18(1–2):35–39.

[50] Kallewaard JW, Vanelderen P, Richardson J, Van Zundert J, Heavner J, Groen GJ. Epiduroscopy for patients with lumbosacral radicular pain. Pain Pract. 2014;14(4):365–77.

[51] Brian Gill J, Heavner JE. Visual impairment following epidural fluid injections and epiduroscopy: a review. Pain Med. 2005;6(5):367–374.

[52] Beyaz SG. Seizures and transient neurological deficits during epiduroscopy in a patient with failed back surgery syndrome. Pain Med. 2015;16(4):825–827.

[53] Manchikanti L, Boswel MV, Singh V, Pampati V, Damron KS, Beyer CD. Prevalence of facet joint pain in chronic spinal pain of cervical, thoracic, and lumbar regions. BMC Musculoskelet Disord. 2004;5(15)

[54] Belozer M, Wang G. Epidural adhesiolysis for the treatment of back pain. Health Technol Assess. 2004;5:1–19.